The Consumption Cl

By Michael Blu

First Edition
Paperback print edition ISBN: 978-1-52010-173-6
Amazon Kindle edition ASIN: B01M3YL4H5

Contents

Section 1 – Introduction

"I make myself rich by making my wants few."
—Henry David Thoreau

BACKGROUND

WHAT'S WRONG WITH CONSUMERISM?

The intention of this book is not to persuade the reader of why our current consumption-based economic and global systems are not healthy. This book picks up where that explanation leaves off. The comprehensive and undeniable explanation of how we got here, how we value money and material possessions over well-being, and how we have become detached from the true measures of a good life has already been told by numerous brave scholars.

This book concerns what happens next. It concerns what happens at the personal level. It is about what I did and what you can do to address consumerism. But I would be remiss if I did not summarise my thoughts about the consumerism problem to provide some context.

William Rees, an urban planner, notes, "It requires four to six hectares of land to maintain the consumption level of the average person from a high-consumption country. The problem is that in 1990, worldwide there were only 1.7 hectares of ecologically productive land for each person."[1]

This massive deficit has to be made up with something, and as such there are two main sources. The first source is your children and your grandchildren and future generations. The resources required to support this unsustainable level of consumption, such as wood, minerals, water, and air, are typically from non-renewable sources. So, what this generation takes does not get replaced. The sources are finite, so the future generations will effectively pay it backwards. The generations to come will look back from their less plentiful world and ask why we did it. The second source is the expropriation of resources by wealthy countries from poor countries through trade, political swindling and corruption, or through military force.

I am not saying that capitalism is bad. Rather, the current, mostly unregulated variety of capitalism causes a deficit in geographical and generational resources. The current economic system dictates that the more things are produced and consumed the better we are doing. The gross domestic product (GDP) has become the holy grail of national success.

The problem with this all-important measurement is that it ignores the future. It ignores any non-monetary positive aspects of life such as happiness, leisure time, and human connection because nothing is consumed by these aspects of well-being. Bhutan recognises this deficiency and so includes kindness, equality, and humanity in a metric called gross national happiness (GNH). Economic and development plans must pass a GNH review based on a GNH impact statement in a way similar to how some countries such as the United States and Australia require an environmental impact statement to be submitted and approved. GDP also ignores the cost to any unfortunate countries or species that get in the way of 'progress'. In fact, this measurement does not consider many of those who pay a price for extraction, production, consumption, and disposal of goods, which add to a nation's GDP. For example, if more people are unhealthy, then more health products are consumed. According to the GDP this is only a good thing. If more environmental disasters occur, this is also a good thing as it generates massive cash flow from the clean-up.

You can see that this measurement is inadequate and misleading.

To change the way that we measure success and to change the system that goes hand-in-hand with that measurement are monumental tasks. Even if it were acknowledged around the globe that it is a self-destructive and dated system that serves fewer and fewer with each generation, it would be some feat to switch to something better. It would certainly mean economic collapse in many countries. But is that better or worse than a straight-up global collapse caused by that same broken economic system?

Environment must trump economy. The economy needs somewhere to exist, doesn't it? The economy has become too central in our lives, and it needs to be replaced with something sustainable. So instead of bemoaning the current system and witnessing its slow and necessary death (with us in it), let us jump ship now. Start living in the new system. The new system is not based on consumption. It is based on genuine well-being, human connection, and community and does its best to get the hell away from the crazy idea that consumerism and a life-long pursuit of money will somehow bring you happiness.

START WITH YOURSELF

In order to start to right the wrongs of consumerism a behavioural examination at a personal level was required. As I have done throughout the Consumption Cleanse, I used myself as the case study. The first step was to accept that I was a part of the system in which I was programmed to work until retirement, earn lots of money, consume lots of stuff, and not think about the damage all this consumption was doing.

Then it was time to align my life with something closer to my true beliefs:

1. Other than those in poverty, riches do not satisfy appetites; they merely expand them.

2. Working to make money just to buy stuff you don't need is nonsense.

3. The consumption-based economy is a broken system.

4. Well-being and wealth should not be measured monetarily.

5. Frugal living and minimalism in themselves are a lot of fun and foster creativity.

6. Creating is more rewarding than consuming.

7. Why buy it when you can borrow it or grow it?

8. Why should anything you do not be fun?

And as I started to put actions into place to underpin these ideas, I found increasingly that I needed to work less. Some basic actions included:

1. I stopped buying useless things and started selling and giving away unnecessary assets and personal effects.

2. I lived the 'reclaim, repurpose, reuse, and recycle' motto.

3. I started growing what food I could instead of buying it.

4. I created an exit plan from my 'work-consume-sleep' cycle focused on exiting my expensive super-consumerist country.

5. I started looking into ways to make a minimal living that would contribute to my alternative view of how the world could be rather than support the current system and my role in it. I focused on contribution and cooperation, not consumption and competition.

6. I started planning the Consumption Cleanse.

When this all went through the wash, I found myself with a one-way ticket out of my country with no belongings except for a few crates of books and memorable trinkets left with my supportive parents, a 15kg bag with all that I needed to survive, and a Frisbee. Fast-forward six months:

1. I live in a small house in Indonesia with my girlfriend.

2. My priority is my health and well-being and that of those close to me. I start my day at whatever hour I choose with meditation and exercise. After this there are no other 'must do' activities. I study languages and write when I feel like it.

3. I eat quite healthily with fresh produce bought daily from the local organic market. My diet is in line with *The Consumption Cleanse*.

4. I practice minimalism. I spend a minimal amount of money and as such do not need a job, let alone one in

the corporate sector. I make a small amount of money from some hobbies that I enjoy. It's enough, and I could never call what I do 'work'.

5. My lifestyle is ever-improving as I find new ways to avoid using money. Sure, sometimes it's not convenient, but I don't need convenience; I have time.

WHAT IS THE MISSION?

I want to influence change at the individual level, for only there can it work. Governments and corporations work in collusion to support the existing system. That is fine, that is their job. But at the risk of sounding subversive, our job if we don't agree with the current system is to undermine it. Undermining happens from...under. It happens with people. Call me anti-establishment if you like, but throughout the course of history progressive change has usually started with the people. It has started in the face of power and in protest against the system of the day. Change is inevitable, and this one is undeniably necessary.

Environmental carnage is by and large at the bloodied hands of consumerism. If the enemy is consumerism and I needed to start with myself, then the logical next step was to reduce my consumption. My plan became to spend a year radically adjusting my life by consuming minimally and thoughtfully and to document it for anyone who might be interested in doing the same.

ABOUT THE BOOK

WHAT IS THE CONSUMPTION CLEANSE?

The Consumption Cleanse is essentially a record of my research and self-experimentation to eliminate unnecessary and harmful consumables from my life, once a week, cumulatively for 52 weeks. It is dissected into four books. The first, this book, is all about 'Food'. Each category is chosen based on my selection criteria below, researched for supporting facts that confirm their unnecessary or harmful nature, and then removed from my life. Sometimes a category comes with an extraction plan, sometimes with viable replacements, and sometimes both. This is documented together with my own experience to be used as a guide when you take on the cleanse.

I encourage you to follow *The Consumption Cleanse* verbatim. I've done the background work. I have been your guinea pig. You will not die. I am not dead. Based on my experience you will live healthier and happier with the only threat of obesity being towards your wallet.

I selected the 52 categories (13 for Book 1—Food) based on the following tests:

1. The extraction, production, consumption, or disposal of the item must be harmful to you, the environment, or both.

2. The item exists largely because of created demand and would be useless in a world that is healthy, happy, and free from the clutches of the dying economic system of today.

3. If the item has any utility, it should have viable alternatives that are not harmful to you or the environment.

WHY FOLLOW THE CONSUMPTION CLEANSE?

Why not do it? But in case that rationale doesn't do it for you, I'll throw you some other reasons to consider:

1. You only need to read one chapter a week over a three-month period for Book 1, in time for your chosen 'Liberation Day' each week.

2. I provide plenty of referenced scientific research that will make you want to stop consuming the items in the cleanse.

3. I provide extraction plans and replacements where appropriate to make your exit as painless as possible.

4. I document my own experience. I am your lab rat. I have done this cleanse and can tell you that I feel great; my wallet is fatter, and my belly is thinner. Prior to leaving my country and prior to the cleanse I weighed 95 kilograms. The last free scales I stepped

on, shortly after the last food item was cleansed, told me I weighed 78 kilograms.

5. As you consume less you will spend less. You will need less money, and therefore you will have less need to work. Perhaps you can get off the hamster wheel altogether, as I did.

6. With all the poisons and toxins that I've removed from my diet, my body feels healthier, and my mind seems sharper. Yes, it is true that I was starting from a low base.

7. Future generations will thank you. Currently, the finite resources we continue to consume at an unsustainable rate will not be available for future generations.

8. You know reducing consumption is the right thing to do.

A friend of mine who was reviewing this book asked me if I really thought that one person's taking on this challenge could make a difference. My answer is that making a difference only happens one person at a time. That's how massive change happens. If you act, people see this, and perhaps someone else will act. The conversation starts to change, inspiration takes hold, and then societal behaviours change. But none of this will happen unless you start with yourself.

Besides, it does not have to be miserable. I am a specialist in having fun. Fun is my main game. Since I started my extraction process from consumerism, I have never had so much fun and been so healthy.

HOW TO DO THE CONSUMPTION CLEANSE

Here are the simple instructions that you need to follow the Consumption Cleanse:

1. Decide to take the challenge and to become healthier and happier almost immediately.

2. Choose a day of the week that will become your Liberation Day, the day you cease consuming the item from that week forward. I chose Saturday and had a lot of fun binging on the item on the Friday night beforehand.

3. As you quit each item you will stay quit of it until the end of the proscribed fifty-two weeks, and I'd say beyond that for most items.

4. Read the chapter for each week in advance of Liberation Day so that you can take any actions you need to prepare, such as stocking up on replacements. This will also prepare you for the extraction plan and any withdrawal symptom remedies, if applicable.

5. Stick to the schedule religiously, so that quitting these consumables becomes a habit in itself.

6. Every chapter represents one week and one item that you will stop consuming. Each chapter is set out in the same way. I describe precisely what it is, how much we earthlings consume of it, why we consume it, why it is bad for us and the planet, and finally I detail the cleanse itself. The cleanse covers extraction methods, replacements, and the benefits to you and the planet.

7. At the end of each chapter is a dashboard that details the actions that need to be taken before and during the week in question. I also include a menu of what to eat and what not to eat.

Throughout the course of your reducing your consumption you are no doubt going to have 'blowouts', by which I mean you might not be able to help yourself. This is fine. It's bound to happen. The main thing to ensure is that the blowout is contained. Don't let it go beyond that day, and don't let it spread to other categories. It may even be beneficial, as with me and coffee, an item in the cleanse.

I recall a particular day when I had been overly ambitious about how much red wine I could drink the night before. I convinced myself that I needed a coffee. I did not need that coffee. After one single espresso (I used to drink five double espressos every day.), I found myself with cold sweats, visibly shaking, my stomach turning, and in a very nervous disposition. I felt awful. It actually vindicated my decision to quit coffee. So, if you do have a blowout, pay attention to how it makes you feel; chances are it won't feel that great, and it will only strengthen your resolve.

Section 2 – The Consumption Cleanse: Food

WEEK 1 - REFINED SUGAR AND ARTIFICIAL SWEETENERS

"Sugar is the next tobacco, without a doubt, and that industry should be scared. It should be taxed just like tobacco and anything else that can, frankly, destroy lives."

— Jamie Oliver

———————

What white powdery drug with worldwide distribution is behind mass addiction and directly and indirectly related to 8 million deaths globally per year? You guessed it: sugar.

Allow me to set the record straight. Sugar itself is not evil. It occurs naturally in many foods. It is adding excess sugar to your dietary intake that is the problem. It's not that medical folks out there are saying that a teaspoon of sugar will strike you down mercilessly in the street, but there is a growing body of research that demonstrates the connection between sugar and obesity. Obesity all by itself isn't a major killer, but heart disease, diabetes, and some cancers (endometrial, breast, colon, kidney, gallbladder, and liver) are, and they are often caused by obesity. On top of that, sugar ingestion can lead to heart disease and diabetes even in people with healthy weights. From many sources, I know that the worldwide deaths from these conditions in 2012 were 23.3 million, including heart disease at 17 million, of which 23% can be attributed to obesity; diabetes at 1.5 million, of which 44% can be attributed to obesity; certain cancers at 2 million, of which between 7% and 41% can be attributed to obesity; and obesity itself 2.8 million.[2] There you have your yearly 8 million deaths from excessive consumption of the crack cocaine of the sweetener world.

WHAT ARE REFINED AND ARTIFICIAL SUGARS?

Stuff just tastes better when it has some sweetness in it. The issues are what we should avoid and what we should use to get this effect while not killing ourselves to get it.

This chapter concerns the adding of sugar and artificial sweeteners to your food and drinks. Because sugar is such a monster topic, food and drinks manufactured with added sugar such as soda and confectionery are covered in separate chapters.

So, let's look at added sugar first. Whether it is raw (cane sugar), white, or brown sugar, all sugar is processed or refined to some degree. To make raw sugar, machines juice the sugar cane, and to that juice lime is added to achieve the desired ph. balance and to rid the resulting liquid of impurities. This is then evaporated and passed through a centrifuge to get sugar crystals, which are then dried further to get the light brown substance known as raw sugar.

To make white sugar, sulphur dioxide is added to bleach the cane juice prior to evaporation. Phosphoric acid, calcium hydroxide, or carbon dioxide is used to remove the impurities from the result, which is then passed through a carbon filter before being crystallised in a vacuum. This is then left to evaporate to get white 'table sugar'. Sounds appetising, doesn't it?

Brown sugar, I was surprised to discover, is even more processed than table sugar. It is, in fact, table sugar mixed with molasses. Inviting molasses to the party does mean that brown sugar contains more nutritional value than white sugar, and so it could be said that it is healthier. But it is akin to saying poking your eye out with a hot iron is okay for you as long as you rub aloe vera on it afterwards. Brown sugar is a source of minimal dietary potassium, calcium, magnesium, and B vitamins but has all of the same negative health effects as table sugar.

In terms of nutritional value, calories, and your body's metabolism, there is no meaningful difference between these types of sugars. But if you simply must eat sugar—though hopefully you won't after reading this—choose raw sugar as it involves fewer processing steps, consumes less energy, uses fewer resources and chemicals, and produces less waste. Surprisingly, brown sugar is the worst choice because it is more processed than white sugar.

Concerning artificial (sugar free) sweeteners, there is a veritable cornucopia of products, all of which should be avoided: Aspartame (Equal, Splenda, and Nutrasweet), acesulfame potassium (Sunett, Ace K), and saccharin (Sweet 'N Low).

The third category of sweetener after sugar and artificial sweeteners is 'natural alternatives', which are not associated with the many negative health effects, including death, like the first two are. These can continue to be consumed in moderation. This category includes raw honey, blackstrap molasses, pure maple syrup, cinnamon (sugar free), stevia (sugar free), and Xylitol (sugar free).

HOW MUCH DO WE CONSUME AND WHY?

Our love for sugar may not at first appear to herald the end of life as we know it, but, in fact, it does bring us closer to that end a lot faster. It has been progressively sneaking its way into our diet so much so that it is now added into 80% of the food sold in supermarkets.[3] It is appearing in increasing amounts and causing a devastating amount of disease and death such that it has overtaken tobacco as a leading cause of death.

Supermarkets are the dealers of the sugar cartels. There is so little healthy sugar free food in supermarkets that it usually takes up less than one aisle and is even labelled for you as 'health food'. For consistency, I'd like to see the other twenty-three and a half aisles labelled 'unhealthy food'.

We are consuming way more sugar than we need. It is delivering abundant human and planetary misery for absolutely no gain whatsoever, given that it has zero nutritional value. "Americans currently consume 22 teaspoons of sugar per day," says Bethany Doerfler, RD, LDN, and a clinical research dietician at Northwestern Medicine in Chicago. That's more than three times as much as what's recommended by the American Heart Association. As for children, the number is actually higher at 32 teaspoons per day. And it is getting worse. In 1900 the United States consumed about five pounds of sugar per person, per year. This skyrocketed to 150 pounds per person by 2000.

The World Health Organisation puts the safe amount of sugar in a healthy diet at no more than 10%, whereas the US sugar industry has claimed that 25% of our diet can safely consist of sugar—a disagreement with an obvious agenda. Companies selling sugary junk know that we drool over sweet stuff, they know how addictive it is, and they know that sugar actually makes consumers consume more (the physiological explanation will come later). It's a win-win for these companies, and it is a lose-lose for people and for the earth. It is an unnecessary consumable that chews up global resources in its growing, processing, marketing, selling, eating, and finally in the health care required to deal with its effects.

————————

If this poison is so bad for us, why are we consuming so damn much of it? The answer is that sugar is addictive. When we consume sugar, dopamine is released into the brain to invoke pleasure. The addict, once hooked, embarks upon the road to obesity and towards a plethora of other health problems. Cravings are real, and because sugar is the crack cocaine of the sweetener world, when we add it to our food and drinks, we need *more*. "Studies are showing that in some people and animals, the brain can react to sugar very much like it can to drugs and alcohol," Doerfler says. That's why when you cut added sugars from your diet, you might feel deprived for a few days. Joel Fuhrman, author of *The End of Dieting*, says, "When your body is overloaded with waste, you feel more uncomfortable when not eating that food. It's like stopping coffee."

As for sugar's chemical compadre, we consume artificial sweeteners because they have the same sweetness we are addicted to and we think that this is a safe way to get our fix. It is not. It is the equivalent of thinking that your addiction is resolved by coming off heroin and jumping on methadone. The important thing to note is that while artificial sweeteners are not sugar and hence have different effects on the body while avoiding some of the negative impacts of sugar, artificial sweeteners come with a whole new raft of health issues.

WHY ARE REFINED AND ARTIFICIAL SUGARS BAD?

Other than its unbeatable addictive qualities, limited nutritional value, and vast swathes of earth that are cleared in order to grow it, why is sugar so bad for us?

First, it is important to note that glucose is actually required by our brains and cells to function. Lactose is primarily in dairy, including mothers' milk, so it follows that this also is required by the body, particularly young bodies. Sucrose, which is half glucose and half fructose, is what makes our food sweet. The primary reason why added sugars are so bad for you is that they contain a large quantity of fructose.

Glucose is essential and can be metabolised by pretty much every cell in the body. If we don't get it from the diet, our bodies make it from proteins and fat. Fructose, however, is not essential to our functioning in any way. Fructose is bad. The only organ that can metabolise fructose is the liver. When large amounts of fructose enter the liver and it is already full of glycogen, most of the fructose gets turned into fat. Some of the fat gets shipped out, but part of it remains in the liver. The fat can build up over time and ultimately lead to non-alcoholic fatty liver disease. This process is the leading cause of obesity, which can lead to diabetes and other related ailments such as high blood pressure and cholesterol. Fructose is present in fruit, but in small quantities and accompanied by plenty of vitamins, minerals, fibre, and water. Also, because it's not easy to overindulge in fruit, fructose from fruit is excluded from this discourse.

Here are the leading reasons you might consider to motivate you to get off refined sugar.[4]

1. **Known cause of non-alcoholic fatty liver disease.** (See above)

2. **Known cause of insulin resistance leading to obesity and type 2 diabetes.** (See above)

3. **Known cause of leptin (hormone) resistance.** Leptin is secreted by our fat cells. The fatter we are the more leptin is secreted. Leptin is supposed to tell the brain we are full and to stop eating. In obese individuals, the response to leptin isn't working right (leptin resistance), so the tendency is to eat more calories than needed. Willpower is no match for a leptin-based starvation signal. To reverse leptin resistance, sugar consumption has to stop.

4. **Known cause of high blood pressure and high cholesterol.** Sugar raises bad cholesterol and

triglycerides and causes various other issues that can ultimately lead to heart disease.

5. **No vitamins or minerals.** Sugar contains only empty calories. Eating high-sugar foods that contain very little nutrients instead of more nutritious foods will likely result in deficiencies of those nutrients.

6. **Not a cause of proper satiety.** Studies show that fructose does not cause satiety like glucose does, which contributes to a higher calorie intake.[5]

7. **Bad choice of land use.** According to *Sistah Vegan*:

> It is 2009, and sugar consumption continues to increase globally. Sucrose is a toxin and has no nutritional value to the human body. Isn't that a little strange? Particularly, since sugar cane is grown upon thousands of acres of land to produce sucrose. Eight hundred and thirty million people in the world are undernourished, and 791 million of them live in so-called developing countries. Hence, what nourishing foods could these acres potentially grow if (a) sugar cane were no longer in high demand from the US (as well as the rest of the top consumers: Brazil, Australia, and the EU) and (b) the land was used specifically to grow nourishing foods for the population in the global South?[6]

As for artificial sweeteners, studies have linked artificial sweeteners to migraines, cancerous tumours, anxiety, and even weight gain amongst other ailments. The June 2010 issue of the *Yale Journal of Biology and Medicine* states that aspartame, acesulfame potassium, and saccharin increase your desire to eat more.

I must confess that from my research, while some tests have been shown to be conclusive in rats, I have been unable to find any conclusive tests that have widespread acceptance about the negative effects of artificial sweeteners on humans. But given that artificial sweeteners are relatively new to the human diet, unless you are drawn to games such as Russian roulette, leave them out of your diet.

THE CLEANSE

Now that the damage that can be caused by sugar and artificial sweeteners has been exposed, the name of the game is to axe sugar from your diet. Because of sugar's drug-like behaviour in the human body, kicking the habit is not as straightforward as simply taking everything in moderation. Alcoholics cannot just have one drink. Cocaine fiends cannot do just one line. The only way to handle such a true physiological addiction is the cold turkey approach. But you won't have to white-knuckle it because if you follow these suggestions, you will be able to reset your body's neurotransmitters and hormones and the sugar-free step will be as painless as possible.

I found this week to be relatively easy as I had not added refined sugar to my homemade food and drinks for some time. It is when I am eating out that I have to be on guard. I didn't realise how common place it was for cafés and restaurants to add sugar to their products, particularly to beverages. I find myself now asking wait staff to please not add sugar to smoothies and juices, for instance. Be alert. Sugar agents are everywhere.

1. **Start the day with protein.** Eat protein at every meal, particularly breakfast, to balance blood sugar and insulin and cut cravings. Eat organic, free-range eggs and protein shakes. Include nuts, seeds, lentils, other high-protein vegetables and fish in moderation in your meals.

2. **Eat plenty of vegetables.** Eat many non-starchy veggies including but not limited to greens, broccoli, cauliflower, kale, collards, asparagus, green beans, mushrooms, onions, zucchini, tomatoes, fennel, eggplant, artichokes, and peppers. Leave out potatoes, sweet potatoes, squash, beets, grains, and beans initially on account of their high carbohydrate content. This will expedite the withdrawal process. After two weeks you will have lost weight and be feeling great. At this time, you can slowly re-introduce those excluded vegetables.

3. **Eat lots of good fats.** Along with protein, eat plenty of good fats at every meal to balance your blood sugar and fuel your cells. Good fats are found in nuts, seeds, extra virgin olive oil, coconut butter, coconut oil, and avocados, and there are omega-3 fats in certain fish (subject to the subsequent chapter on seafood).

4. **Pack healthy snacks.** Whether you're at home, at work, or on the road, keep ration packs of healthy snacks on hand to dig into when you feel the need to consume sugar. Snacks can include any of the ingredients mentioned above. This can be something as simple as a trail mix of nuts and seeds that you can graze on instead of snack food at airports, fish jerky that you can whip out when

you are drawn to a confectionery machine, canned fish or oysters that you can unpeel at a moment's notice, and any other favourite made from protein, good carbs, and fats.

5. **Avoid inflammation.** Studies show that inflammation triggers blood sugar imbalances, insulin resistance, pre-diabetes, and type 2 diabetes. The most common source of inflammatory foods other than sugar, flour, and trans fats are hidden food sensitivities, most commonly gluten and dairy. Stay away from gluten for the same two weeks as with the excluded vegetables above. You'll notice a difference in you energy levels and cravings, and if you have symptoms of intolerance, they should disappear in this time as well. Note that subsequent chapters deal more comprehensively with gluten and dairy.

6. **Get enough sleep.** Not getting sufficient sleep causes sugar and carbohydrate cravings by affecting your appetite hormones. Studies have shown that humans deprived of two hours of the recommended eight hours of sleep per night experienced increases in hunger hormones, decreases in appetite-suppressing hormones, and increases in cravings for sugar and refined carbohydrates.

7. **Use natural alternatives.** When something absolutely, positively needs to be made sweeter, use one of the natural alternatives to sugar. When you have a choice between something sweetened with processed sugar and something sweetened by a natural alternative, choose the latter.

———————

There is no need to add refined sugar and artificial sweeteners in your food and beverages when there are loads of natural alternatives. Natural alternatives deliver the sweetness that you seek and add their unique flavour and health benefits.

1. **Raw honey.** Raw honey is packed full of flavonoids and antioxidants that reduce the risk of heart disease and some cancers along with vitamins, minerals, and enzymes that help boost your immune system and protect your body from bacteria. Honey also has a low hypoglycaemic index that will help reduce blood sugar spikes. Generally speaking, the most nutrient-dense honeys are the darker varieties.

2. **Blackstrap molasses.** Molasses is a by-product of sugarcane processing and contains high levels of iron, calcium, copper, and manganese. It has a toasty, slightly bitter flavour and high levels of antioxidants.

3. **Pure maple syrup.** Packed full of polyphenols, a plant-based compound that works as an antioxidant, maple syrup also helps with muscle recovery because it is a source of manganese, a mineral used in the muscle recovery process. It also contains zinc, iron, calcium, and potassium and is a great alternative to use for baking.

4. **Cinnamon (sugar free).** My personal favourite, cinnamon is not only plant based and completely sugar free, it also tastes great. You can use cinnamon sticks or powder, but be wary of some cinnamon powders as they are blended with refined sugar. Can you believe sugar has even infiltrated its own alternatives? Cinnamon helps to reduce sugar cravings by controlling blood glucose levels by minimising insulin spikes after meals. It has also been

shown to lower LDL-cholesterol and triglyceride blood levels. Ceylon cinnamon is the true form of cinnamon, and it is widely considered the best for blood sugar control and losing weight.

5. **Stevia (sugar free).** Stevia is a sweet-tasting natural herb commonly used in tea, coffee, and desserts. This natural sweetener extracted from the leaves of the stevia plant contains several nutrients including phosphorus, calcium, proteins, vitamins, magnesium, zinc, and sodium. Make sure your stevia product does not contain maltodextrin, dextrose, or any other sugar derivative.

6. **Xylitol (sugar free).** Sugar alcohols such as xylitol, sorbitol, and erythritol are natural sweeteners that contain fewer calories than refined sugar, about two calories per gram on average. Refined sugar contains four calories per gram. While sugar alcohols can raise your blood sugar level, they won't affect your blood sugar as much as other sugars because your body doesn't completely absorb sugar alcohols. The Mayo Clinic warns that when eaten in large amounts, typically more than 50 grams, they can have a laxative effect.

Coconut palm sugar or syrup, a common natural alternative, is not included in this list due to environmental concerns. Once the sap is extracted for its sugar, the plant does not produce coconuts anymore. For coconut production to remain the same, it would be necessary to cultivate more land or reduce coconut consumption to obtain more coconut palm sugar.

Also avoid sweeteners derived from palm oil. Living in Indonesia has opened my eyes to the massive devastation to the forests and its inhabitants at the hands of the rapid expansion of palm oil plantations.

————

Giving up sugar and artificial sweeteners must surely be compelling by this point. Other than there being less likelihood of collecting any number of the ailments mentioned above, the advantages below are just your icing (sugar-free of course) on the cake.

1. **You'll stop wanting sugar.** Once you have removed processed sugar from your diet and resolved your addiction, you will gradually lose the desire to eat anything with processed sugar in it. When you do, the blood sugar spike and subsequent comedown will reinforce why you decided to stop consuming it.

2. **You will consume less.** When sugar is taken out of your diet, for the reasons explained above, you will consume less, and the earth will thank you.

3. **Your energy will increase.** We tend to think that sugar-filled foods such as energy drinks are what we need to boost energy, but in fact sugar blocks your body's ability to keep your energy levels optimised. Without this sugar you would have a higher energy level naturally without the steep peaks and troughs in your blood sugar levels causing you to crash once the effects of the sugar rush wear off.

4. **You will lose weight.** Sugar and sugary food make you crave more of whatever it is in, which often is high in

carbohydrates, processed or junk food, and drink. On top of sugar, these poor excuses for food probably have loads of other ingredients that are not good for you. By walking away from sugar you won't need to deal with all of those extra calories; you will feel less hungry and will almost certainly shed excess weight.

5. **Your gut will function more efficiently.** By eliminating processed sugar you are allowing your stomach and bowels (and other internal organs) to behave more naturally when processing what you have eaten. In one recent study sugar was shown to promote the growth of bad gut bacteria.[7]

6. **Your skin will look better.** Sugar may be affecting your skin from the inside. Many people report that their skin looks and feels healthier after they have quit sugar.

As my only sugar eradication effort involved times when I was eating and drinking out, this week did not pose much of a challenge for me, but it did feel satisfying to know that I was finally a hard-line anti-sugar preacher. Things were a bit tougher quitting confectionery, as covered in a later chapter.

One thing I did not expect was how much I could taste the ingredients in my smoothies and juices. Sugar had been homogenising them to such a degree that now I found myself choosing different ingredients because the old ones didn't taste like I thought they did.

ACTIONS

•Watch Damon Gameau's, *That Sugar Film*
http://www.thatsugarfilm.com/film.

•Stock up on sugar replacements so your sweet tooth has fewer options.

•Quit adding refined sugar to food and drinks on Liberation Day.

•Save yourself from a life full of sugar-related health issues.

MENU

Do Eat	Eat in Moderation	Eat If You Must	Do Not Eat
Cinnamon, Stevia	Raw Honey, Blackstrap Molasses, Pure Maple Syrup & Xylitol	Coconut Palm Sugar or Syrup	Raw (Cane), White or Brown Sugar Artificial Sweeteners Sweeteners Derived from Palm Oil

WEEK 2 -BEER

"Give a man a beer, waste an hour. Teach a man to brew, and waste a lifetime!"

—Bill Owen

————————

I exist because of beer. Some archaeologists claim that our ancestors, the first farmers back in the Stone Age around 11,500 years ago, actually started growing cereals to make booze, not food. Folks back then would go to great efforts to obtain and cultivate grains to be processed into beer's Neolithic relative. That's what I call priorities!

With the domestication of cereals came the advent of agriculture, one of the great evolutionary leaps of mankind. I choose to believe that the nudge forwards that beer gave us is why we are here today. I drink beer; therefore, I am.

With such acclaim and knowing that my very existence is thanks to beer, why am I turning my back on it? Before you turn off your Kindle in disgust, unsubscribe, or unfriend me on Facebook, let me explain. I love beer. I think it's fantastic. I think beer likes me too—a lot. It is, or rather was, my tipple of choice. At the end of a hot summer's day, after a long day at work, or at a sporting event, there are not many times that don't call for a refreshing ale. I confess that I also enjoy beer in winter, in the morning, and whilst not at sporting events. I have consumed glorious beer for my entire adult life, mostly by force of habit. It was my default beverage.

So why, then? This book is all about disruption, especially this chapter. I was drinking beer on autopilot, usually piling up the empty vessels without a great deal of conscious brain activity. I could blame the ancestors and my genome, but the reality is that this was a consumption habit that I had developed unassisted. So to make the decision to consume stuff or not a conscious one, to derail the beer train, nothing short of abstinence was required. I anticipated that I would consume less alcohol in general. I hoped the cleanse would remove whatever reliance I had on it, freeing me from one more unnecessary vice. I could always choose to re-insert it into my diet after a year.

Ultimately, this book is not about removing fun from your life. Alcohol is fun. So, I will continue to consume all other alcoholic beverages except beer. In this chapter, I ignore any positive health aspects of beer. I discuss only the negatives to make myself feel better about giving it up. If you do not like beer, I suggest you substitute your alcoholic beverage of choice. Stop drinking whatever beverage will shake your tree the most.

WHAT IS IT?

Beer . . . is beer.

On the unlikely chance that you do not know what beer is, Wikipedia's "Beer" page tells us:

Beer is the world's most widely consumed and likely the oldest alcoholic beverage; it is the third most popular drink overall, after water and tea. The production of beer is called brewing, which involves the fermentation of starches, mainly derived from cereal grains—most commonly malted barley, although wheat, maize (corn), and rice are widely used.

It also tastes great.

How Much Do We Consume and Why?

It should come as no surprise that the global brewing business is dominated by a handful of multinational conglomerates. There are also thousands upon thousands of smaller operations ranging from brewpubs and craft beer operations all the way down to the one-man band, the home brewer. Globally, around 150 billion litres of beer are sold each year.

In terms of who is doing all the drinking, the Europeans, in particular in the Czech Republic, are the biggest consumers per capita by a country mile. The top fifteen countries by consumption per capita are shown below.[8]

Rank	Country	Consumption per capita [1] (litres)	2013–2014 change (633–ml bottles)	Total national consumption $(10^6 L)^{[A]}$	Year
1	Czech Republic	142.6	-7.3	1879	2014
2	Seychelles	114.6	7.8	11	2014
3	Austria	104.8	-1.7	894	2014
4	Germany	104.7	4.4	8441	2014
5	Namibia	104	-7.2	250	2014
6	Poland	97.8	0.1	3776	2014
7	Ireland	97	-0.5	454	2014
8	Lithuania	96.6	10.7	282	2014
9	Belize	93.8	-8.8	33	2014
10	Estonia	93.5	-5	123	2014
11	Gabon	88.9	22.3	150	2014
12	Romania	85.9	8.3	1689	2014
13	Spain	80.6	5.9	3729	2014
14	Finland	78.5	-2.7	430	2014
15	Latvia	78.2	4.6	156	2014

And the Czechs make some tasty beers. Another interesting fact I came across was the location of the highest density of breweries in the world. The German Region of Franconia, especially in the district of Upper Franconia, has about 200 breweries, most of them microbreweries. I best stop this line of discussion for fear of a blowout, but I know where I'm going in twelve months.

————————

Why we consume beer is by and large part of a bigger question: "Why do we consume alcohol?" Perhaps just because it's fun. It is also consumed as part of habits and rituals. It can be a social lubricant or crutch and can also be addictive. These reasons all apply to beer as well, but I'm not here to talk about the complex topic of alcohol; I will focus on the reasons that we drink beer specifically.

One idea swilling about in my mind is that we drink beer because we have always drunk beer. After so many generations from 11,500 years ago when those ancient party animals first made beer, it may well have become part of our genetic makeup to like beer. Aside from that wild assumption, beer has a relatively low alcohol content per ounce compared to wine and spirits so more of it can be consumed making it a suitable social drink. It is relatively cheap and refreshing, and there's the beer-buzz you just don't get from other drinks. Most consumers would agree that it is an acquired taste, and once acquired, it is hard to dispose of.

WHY IS BEER BAD?

The following, again, deals only with beer, not with drinking alcohol in general.

1. **Ingredients.** I was surprised to learn that in a lot of the Western countries I examined, beer companies were not required by law to declare the ingredients in their brews on their packaging. They lobby hard to keep this the case for good reason. Many of the massive beer conglomerates have been found to put all sorts of crap in their beer. They certainly aren't held to a standard such as the beer purity laws in Germany. There, the only ingredients that can be used in the production of beer are water, barley, and hops. After its discovery, yeast too was added to the law. Indeed, it would seem that the largest beer companies are

no longer producing beer, but its mutant cousin. To cut costs and encourage more consumption, many high-selling beers contain MSG, high fructose corn syrup, propylene glycol, hop extract instead of real hops, artificial colouring (too bad if you have allergies), GMO corn and animal products like fish bladders and insect-based dyes (too bad if you are a vegetarian—which you might well be after you read the Land-Based Animals chapter).

2. **Gluten**. Typically, beer contains malted barley, which contains gluten. Some folks are sensitive to gluten, particularly those with Celiac disease, where gluten triggers the immune system into attacking the lining of the small intestine.

3. **Beer belly**. Alcohol in general causes weight gain, but beer most of all. Beer contains very little nutrition for its 140–200 calories in a typical bottle. Light beer is less at a hundred calories. Beer also encourages you to eat more. It interferes with your liver's ability to convert glycogen into glucose. When blood sugar drops and your liver doesn't create glucose, your body thinks it is hungry, and you will eat the most readily accessible foods. When you're drinking beer, you don't exactly feel like eating an alfalfa and bamboo shoot salad. You want pizza or a greasy kebab. Don't ask me why, but it's true.

4. **UDIs**. Unidentified drinking injuries are common, especially for beer drinkers. I am basing this not on any documented research but based on more than twenty-five years of self-experimentation. I don't know how these happen; they are unidentified.

5. **Hydration**. Who doesn't love a cold beer when you're hot? But it could be a bad idea. Anti-diuretic hormones

help your body retain fluid. Alcohol interferes with this hormone's release, which explains those frequent bathroom visits when drinking beer. With all that liquid on the way out, hydration can be an issue.

6. **False strength**. Drinking too much beer can make some people think they are a lot stronger than they really are. Injuries are often caused by beer drinkers' attempting feats requiring non-existent super-human strength.

Globally, beer does not have a particularly devastating impact on the environment, but everything we consume has some impact. A bigger carbon footprint is associated with distance travelled and packaging. If you're drinking imported beer instead of a tasty local craft beer, your environmental impact will be more significant. The CO_2 footprint of some common beer-swilling approaches are:

300g CO2e: locally brewed cask ale at the pub.

500g CO2e: local bottled beer from a shop or foreign beer in a pub.

900g CO2e: bottled beer from the shop, extensively transported.

If you drink local beer at the ale house instead of imported beer in a bottle at home, then you're doing your bit for the environment.

THE CLEANSE

The idea in this chapter is to break a consumption habit. The habit to break is not all alcohol, heaven forbid, but your favourite habitual drink. Mine was beer, and that's a good one to stop drinking based on the ill effects described above. You need to consciously not buy your usual alcoholic beverage and consciously buy something else. Hopefully, when the act of buying a drink is conscious, you will not only appreciate it more, you'll be breaking an old habit and drink something healthier.

If you want to drink the same amount of alcohol as you did previously, go right ahead, I do. My replacement beverage is red wine. I was already a red wine drinker; so now I drink wine when I would normally drink wine, and I also drink wine when I would normally drink beer. So many antioxidants! If you replace it with spirits, remember that white spirits are generally less bad for you than dark spirits, and you need to think hard about a mixer, as soft drinks come off the menu in this cleanse. Neat tequila, perhaps?

You might notice as I did that regular activities that previously involved guzzling beer now take on a new light. Guzzling wine instead delivers a different type of buzz, and you know what they say, 'Change is as good as a holiday'.

––––––––

Your choice of replacement beverage is entirely up to you, of course. Alcohol is not good for you regardless of what it is, so do what you can to pick a healthier option than beer. I find it hard to go past red wine when I'm looking for the least unhealthy way to get on the drip. In fact, red wine in moderation is increasingly touted as being good for you in the following ways.

1. **Heart.** The flavonoids and saponins in red wine help protect you against cardiovascular disease.

2. **Resveratrol.** The resveratrol in wine helps clear the saturated fat clogging up your arteries, reduces skin crinkles and lines, and helps slow the ageing process in general. Red wine makes you young again.

3. **Weight loss.** Researchers at the Oregon State College of Agricultural Studies took a closer look at the benefits of red wine and found that ellagic acids inside of a pinot noir grape can delay the growth of fat cells and slow the development of new ones.[9] In the experiment, the mice drinking pinot, aside from notably having a better time, stored less liver fat than did the sober mice, and they had lower blood sugar.

4. **Cancer.** Red wine helps reduce the chance of breast and lung cancer.

5. **Dementia.** It also helps reduce the risk of dementia and Alzheimer's disease.

6. **Sleep.** I'm not referring to drinking until you pass out. It's the melatonin in red wine that helps you sleep easier.

7. **Teeth.** Red wine hardens teeth enamel, slowing tooth decay. It also can reduce gum inflammation and prevent gum diseases.

8. **Replaces workouts**. I love this one. Researchers at the University of Alberta in Canada showed that resveratrol in red wine can benefit our health in the same way as a one-hour workout.[10] I don't know about you, but hitting the bar for an hour of high-impact red wine drinking or going to the park for some interval red wine drinking sounds pretty good to me.

———————

The main conundrum that I faced with the beer week was that it most probably was not going to have much positive influence on the environment. You most likely will replace beer with something else, so the net effect could be nil. You can make a small difference, however by buying locally, whatever your poison may be, and minimising packaging. The big gains to be had here are personal.

In my case—and let's face it, this is my book—weight loss and the list of health benefits associated with my replacement drink accounted for the first part of the personal gain. I lost loads of weight throughout the cleanse, and while I cannot categorically attribute a specific amount of that to my not drinking beer, I know that it is so. I now drink a lot less than I did as I no longer have all-night beer-drinking sessions. And thanks to the melatonin in wine, sleep kicks in now before I become a hazard to myself.

The second personal benefit is a bit more sublime. Being able to break a life-long bad habit and put the controls back in my hands have meant that when I drink, I consciously decide what and how much. Each drink is a conscious decision, not an automatic action. I think there's something in that.

So, in closing, we raise a toast of thanks but no thanks to Ninkasi, the Mesopotamian goddess of beer, as we say to her, "Nice knowing you, but good-bye for now".

ACTIONS

• Decide what your replacement beverage will be.

• Quit drinking beer on Liberation Day.

• Enjoy a new kind of buzz and watch your beer belly contract.

MENU

Do Drink	Drink in Moderation	Drink If You Must	Do Not Drink
Water, water and more water	Red wine	Other alcoholic beverages	Beer (or your favourite tipple if you do not drink beer)

WEEK 3 - CONFECTIONERY

"Oom pa loom pa doom pa dee doo.

I've got a perfect puzzle for you.

Oom pa loom pa doom pa dee dee.

If you are wise, you'll listen to me.

What do you get when you guzzle down sweets?

Eating as much as an elephant eats.

What are you at getting terribly fat?

What do you think will come of that?

I don't like the look of it!

Oom pa loom pa doom pa dee dah.

If you're not greedy, you will go far.

You will live in happiness too,

Like the oom pa loom pa doompadee do!

Doom pa dee doo!"

—Charlie and the Chocolate Factory, by Roald Dahl

———————

45

Have you seen *Willy Wonka & the Chocolate Factory* (1971), based on the 1964 book written by Roald Dahl, *Charlie and the Chocolate Factory*? It is a vastly popular film, a fantasy of such sugary proportions that simply watching it raises your risk of type 2 diabetes. That said, Willy Wonka's factory has more in common with a health farm managed by Saint Theresa (may she rest in peace) than with the deceptive and destructive real world of modern-day confectionery.

At this point in the cleanse, you have already stopped consuming processed sugar. However, its most common and profligate outlet is confectionery, so it too must go as part of this cleanse. Sugar is sugar regardless of whether it is pure or bundled in with a whole bunch of other nasty stuff and called 'sweets'. All of the negative health effects detailed in the Refined Sugar and Artificial Sweeteners chapter are applicable, and so I won't belabour them here.

Instead, this chapter's focus is on what you are supporting when you buy confectionery. The aim is to provide a compelling case to persuade you to boycott the gigantic multinational confectionery cartels. It is not only because the junk they produce is bad for you, completely unnecessary in the human diet, and devastating for the planet, but also because of the ruthless and deceitful way in which they conduct business.

Whether it is child labour, misleading labelling, unethical promotion, environmental catastrophe, pollution or price fixing, your purchasing of confectionery is enabling it. The bottom line? Confectionery must go.

WHAT IS IT?

From Wikipedia:

Confectionery is the art of making confections, which are food items that are rich in sugar and carbohydrates. Exact definitions are difficult. In general, though, confectionery is divided into two broad and somewhat overlapping categories: bakers' confections and sugar confections.

Bakers' confectionery, also called flour confections, includes principally sweet pastries, cakes, donuts and similar baked goods.

Sugar confectionery includes sweets, candied nuts, chocolates, chewing gum, sweetmeats, pastillage, and other confections that are made primarily of sugar. (...) The words candy (US and Canada), sweets (UK and Ireland), and lollies (Australia and New Zealand) are common words for the most common varieties of sugar confectionery.

Not specifically mentioned in the Wikipedia definition but included this week for termination are ice cream and sugared breakfast cereals. Including breakfast cereal here might surprise you. Sugared breakfast cereals are some of the most commonly consumed processed foods that have added sugars. Anything with added sugar or artificial sweeteners including HFCS and Molitol, the industry's latest attempt at deception about this subcategory of junk food, is now on the chopping block. HFCS is well studied and known to be exceptionally bad for you. Molitol is relatively new, but there are as many studies claiming ill effects as there are those claiming it is benign. So don't risk it. Besides, boycotting Big Confectionery is reason enough to get off this poor excuse for food.

These foods can be identified by reading the ingredients list on the labels of the products. Generally, the list of ingredients is ordered according to the quantity of each ingredient in the product in descending order. If you see these ingredients listed early in the list, you know there is plenty of it crammed in there.

Alternatively, you can familiarise yourself with the large multinational companies that produce this junk food and boycott them. I'll name and shame some of the big offenders. It seems that Nestlé takes the cake (pun intended) in terms of global miscreants, but it is joined by others such as Mars, Kraft Foods, Cadbury, and Hershey's. The central strategy of these bad boys is to get you on the drip and keep you there until addiction, obesity, and death do you part.

How Much Do We Consume and Why?

We may know that sugary confectionery is not good for our physiological systems. So why the devil are we drawn to it? Well folks, we are drawn to it because of the devil. I am not a religious fellow, but if I were I'd say there was certainly something satanic about these confectionery companies. Willy Wonka in a cameo appearance as the Grim Reaper peddles well-disguised poisons to the addicts on his teat through a number of nasty tactics.

Relentless and unconscionable promotion by Big Confection—such as the highly unethical and deadly Nestlé campaign to promote their baby formula in third world countries (discussed below)—is one way they strive to expand sales. While this is not a confectionery product, it is a confectionery company, and it exposes the extent to which they will go to acquire more addicts.

Intentionally misleading labelling is another favourite. Big Confection is continuously finding new ways to relabel, rebrand, and misinform the population to conceal the truth about these products. Here are some of those methods:

1. **'Low fat', 'reduced fat', and 'fat free'.** No doubt you have seen food labels on confectionery splashing these claims about. Foods that have their fat removed generally taste like plasterboard, not high on taste bud excitement. For this reason, these foods need to be loaded with sugar, artificial sweeteners, and all manner of ungodly chemicals to get people to eat them.

2. **Sugar by many names.** Confectionery manufacturers will often put different types of sugar in their junk food. A product might contain sugar, HFCS syrup, Molitol, rice syrup and evaporated cane juice–all sugar. In this way the volume of each individual type of sugar will be less and subsequently appear further down on the ingredients list where it may not be noticed. Ingredient lists are not usually known for a holding the reader's attention.

3. **More than one serving.** The real sugar quantity is frequently disguised by saying on the packaging that the product contains more than one serving. In my days now past of confectionery eating, I don't recall ever eating just

half of a chocolate bar, even after acknowledging the serving size. I will eat how much I want, and this is usually all of it. Big Confectionery uses this to report less sugar 'per serving.

4. **"All natural'.** The verbal trickery of the food industry strikes again. The term 'natural' suggests the food is free from pesticides and genetically modified organisms (GMOs). Without much labelling regulation, 'all natural' foods usually contain pesticide-sprayed GMO corn, soy, canola, and sugar beets.

The main reason confectionery is consumed and why it continues to grow in distribution and volume is its addictive qualities. From the Refined Sugar and Artificial Sweeteners chapter we know how addictive this ingredient is. It has been proven to create addiction on both a biochemical and neurological level. What is even more sinister here is that Big Confection has been well aware of this all along and, in fact, uses this quality as a central strategy for growth. Their junk food is specifically designed to bypass the appetite control and the neurological security valves of the addict. In the book *Salt, Sugar, Fat: How the Food Giants Hooked Us,*[11] Michael Moss explains that these companies invest enormous amounts of money trying to find the right combinations of the cheapest and most addictive ingredients to put in their junk foods.

The scariest part is yet to come. The addiction to confection is passed on genetically from mother to child. Recent research shows that food choices during pregnancy have an impact on the offspring's food choices. If the mother eats high-sugar junk food, then this also becomes the baby's preference. And what's even more worrisome is that this is not a behavioural inheritance; it is genetic. The DNA and the genes that encode opioid and dopamine receptors in the child's brain are altered such that addiction is more likely.

Eleni Roumeliotou, a geneticist with a master's degree in human molecular genetics, surmises brilliantly:

In a twisted way, the new generation is genetically pre-programmed to be addicted to junk food, even before they are born. This perfect self-feeding loop guarantees long-term profits for the food corporations and chronic debilitating disease for humans, for generations to come. By designing and selling addictive, low quality and disease-promoting products, Big Food has achieved the unthinkable: to create a dedicated army of health-compromised, addicted fans, whose cognitive, biochemical and even genetic potential to break free of their addiction is hijacked before birth.[12]

WHY IS CONFECTIONERY BAD?

Consuming sugar-based confectionery is bad for you primarily because of the sugar and artificial sweeteners that they are loaded up with. Addiction, obesity, diabetes, and a raft of other ailments are coming your way in the not-too-distant future should you not kick this habit and eliminate it from your diet. The odds are against you though, as the addiction has probably made its way into your genetic code, as discussed above, and the Big Confectionery companies will stop at nothing to keep you hooked. You must persist, get off the ride, and withdraw your support for these good-for-nothing profit machines. Do it for you, the next generation, and the planet.

What harm do these ruthless companies cause? I'm glad you asked. Here is a list of some of the more callous global offences I have come across.

1. **Unethical promotion**. Nestlé aggressively promoted its baby formula in the late 70's in a number of third world countries specifically targeting the poor. They pushed their product as something as good as mother's milk and encouraged parents to get off the natural method in order to beef up their bottom line. Sadly, their product did little to beef up the baby. Some of these victims had no access to clean water, were not literate in English, and hence did not boil their polluted water as per the instructions written in English. Nestlé appears to have knowingly ignored these conditions as breastfeeding was cast aside. UNICEF estimates that a formula-fed child living in disease-ridden and unhygienic conditions is between six and twenty-five times more likely to die of diarrhoea and four times more likely to die of pneumonia than a breastfed child.[13]
The International Baby Food Action Network (IBFAN) says that Nestlé distributed free baby formula to hospitals and maternity wards. After leaving the hospital, the families found that the formula was no longer free, but because the lactation process of the mother had been interrupted the baby was stuck on the formula and the family had to continue to pay for it. Ruthless! It is not on the public record exactly how many infants perished from malnutrition and disease because they were not fed mother's milk, but you can be sure there were plenty. Nestlé's response was that something should

be done about the water quality in these places and used that for a platform to sell their bottled water!

2. **Misleading labelling**. GMOs and traces of the industrial poison melamine are used in Nestlé products.[14] Even if you believe the scientists on the Nestlé payroll when they say GMOs are perfectly good for you, melamine is a poison. It sickened 50,000 Chinese infants in 2008.[15] Purina, a subsidiary of Nestlé, is currently in the courts for using propylene glycol, a component of antifreeze and known animal toxin in its dog food. Over 3,000 dogs fell ill, to which Purina responded that propylene glycol is "an FDA-approved food additive that is also in human foods like salad dressing and cake mix".[16] Oh. OK. That's fine then.

3. **Price fixing.** The Canadian Competition Bureau raided the offices of Nestlé Canada, Hershey Canada, Inc., and Mars Canada, Inc., seeking evidence for their price-fixing investigation. Under a class action lawsuit, without admitting liability, these companies settled for a $9 million payout. If corporations could have a conscience, theirs would be a guilty one. In addition, the CEO of Nestlé Canada is facing criminal charges for price fixing.

4. **Environmental damage.** Bottled water and palm oil are two of the consumables behind massive environmental catastrophes perpetrated by, you guessed it, Nestlé. Nestlé is the world's biggest producer of bottled water, a fact underpinned by their Chairman's belief that water should not be a universal right. Chairman Peter Brabeck-Letmathe says: "There are two different opinions on the matter [of water]. The one opinion, which I think is extreme, is represented by the NGOs, who bang on about declaring water a public right. That means that as a

human being you should have a right to water. That's an extreme solution." Is it really, Peter? Then why has your company been pillaging water from California's San Bernardino National Forest without a permit since 1988 and now during one of California's worst droughts in history?[17] An independent analysis puts the usage at 1 billion gallons per year while the rest of the state faces severe restrictions.[18] Then there's the tiny Pakistani village of Bhati Dilwan where Nestlé's deep well deprives locals of potable water. Children are being sickened by the filthy water that remains available to them. "The water is not only very dirty, but the water level sank from 100 to 300 to 400 feet," says a local elder.[19] They can't pipe fresh water in because that would detract from Nestlé's source of profit from their Pure Life brand. And as if this type of environmental and community wreckage were not enough, you've also got their bottling of tap water and labelling it as something else, something for which current lawsuits have been filed against them. Nestlé's Kit Kat brand has been involved in the ongoing palm oil disaster whereby huge tracts of rain forest and their inhabitants, most notably the endangered orang-utans, are destroyed to produce palm oil. It should be noted that Nestlé has ceased sourcing this ingredient in this way, but only after massive people-power protests succeeded.

5. **Child labour, abuse, and trafficking.** *The Dark Side of Chocolate*,[20] a 2010 documentary by Miki Mistrati and U. Roberto Romano, exposed child labour practises in the cocoa plantations on the Ivory Coast. The child slaves were often shipped from nearby countries and were as young as twelve years old. The International Labor Rights Fund sued Nestlé on behalf of three Malian children, claiming they were trafficked to the Ivory Coast, forced to

work as slaves, and beaten regularly. In 2010, the US District Court for the Central District of California determined corporations cannot be held liable for violations of international law and dismissed the suit. This has since been appealed.

6. **Animal Testing.** Nestlé, which makes Nestea, conducts and pays others to conduct painful and deadly tea tests on animals. The company causes animals to suffer simply to investigate the possible health benefits linked to tea products and ingredients, even though not one of these experiments is legally required for beverage manufacturers and regulators have stated that animal tests are not sufficient to prove health claims about food and beverage products. In these cruel tests, mice and rats have been tormented and then killed by decapitation and other methods. See the NesteaCrueltea.com website for further details of the horrors endured by the animals used in Nestea's tea experiments

That's a list long enough for several death sentences if the 'perp' were civilians. You can't execute a corporation, but you can starve it to death by starving it of its food—revenue.

THE CLEANSE

The starting point in giving up confectionery, folks, is to know and identify exactly what it is you are giving up. Hopefully, some of the tips above will give you a better chance of a positive identification of these villains and then the same tactics employed in the Refined Sugar and Artificial Sweeteners chapter will also help you here.

Again, it is a matter of going cold turkey, knowing when you are susceptible to purchasing and eating this junk, and making sure you have good alternatives on hand that you can tuck into. Coming from someone who was quite prone to scoffing down a chocolate bar or two or an ice cream on a fairly regular basis, this week provided me with a view of exactly how much I was consuming in this category. It was loads! I realised that while I wasn't adding sugar to anything, I was consuming it day in and day out. By the end of the week I realised that my small-talk relationships with a vast number of convenience store and take-away shop attendants were over.

Eating better and a good education are the best weapons against the corporate stranglehold that has us eating toxic non-food all the way to the hospital ward.

————

I love chocolate. Eating it is one of the fundamental joys in my life. This cleanse is not about forbidding yourself all the nice things in life; it is about avoiding consumption that has unsustainable impacts on yourself and the world. So I have allowed myself these alternatives to the crap peddled by Big Confectionery that I think still fit within the bounds of what this cleanse is all about.

1. **Dark chocolate.** Dark chocolate, ideally 80% cocoa or more and with natural sugar alternatives for sweetener produced by other than Big Confectionery and ideally

approved by international fair-trade organisations such as Fair Trade.

2. **Fruit and nuts.** Nuts, seeds and berries of all varieties and snacks made from these. Fruit is a good alternative too. Where possible, buy locally grown, or better yet, grow your own.

3. **Raw and rolled oats**. In my wanderings though the breakfast cereal aisles, this consistently turns up as the only breakfast cereal that is not jam-packed with added sugar

I've found that I have some new favourites, only a small collection of very specific dark chocolates that I seek out if I find myself in the sugary aisles of a supermarket. I've also tracked down some boutique chocolate vendors who have a great range of dark chocolate and dark chocolate covered fruit and nuts of which I have become a fan. Other than this I don't eat any sweets, and I assure you the impact on my daily energy level has been immense.

––––––––

I've realised that while I never used to notice the sugar energy spikes from sweets, I definitely noticed the come-downs. These are now gone. My energy level throughout the day is higher than before, and even within the space of one week it seemed I became a bit thinner around my now somewhat less rotund belly.

The other minor impact is that I have saved the equivalent of around $30 AUD a week, which would be about $1,500 a year. Woo hoo!

Once you have removed confectionery from your diet, not only will the positive impacts outlined in the Refined Sugar and Artificial Sweeteners chapter be more pronounced, but you will have pulled support from the companies that really couldn't give a damn for the planet and its inhabitants.

ACTIONS

- Watch the documentary ***The Dark Side of Chocolate***
https://www.youtube.com/watch?v=7Vfbv6hNeng.

- Ensure you have confectionery replacements on hand to combat temptation.

- Quit eating confectionery on Liberation Day.

- Save your teeth, your belly, and your wallet in the process.

MENU

Do Eat	Eat in Moderation	Eat If You Must	Do Not Eat
Fruit-, nut-, and seed-based snacks Raw and rolled oats	Dark chocolate with 80% cocoa and a natural sweetener	Low sugar content breakfast cereals	Bakery and sugar confectionery Ice cream Sugary breakfast cereals

WEEK 4 - SODA AND BOTTLED DRINKS

"Have a Coke and smile."

—1976 Coca Cola marketing slogan

—————

May I suggest that if you drink Coke that you do not smile and do not show your fangs. The research suggests that unless you think folks want to see a mouth that resembles the keys on a synthesiser after an encounter with a mechanical meat separator, remain tightly lipped, please.

How one of the most successful marketing companies in history didn't think that one through, I do not know. It's akin to promoting crystal methamphetamine with "Show 'em your track marks". What's wrong with "Enjoy Coke, but for god's sake don't bare your teeth", or a completely honest promotion? (I do know that is not how the world works.) How about, "Enjoy Coke and enjoy an early death from some obesity-related disease. PS. Make sure you leave some money aside for your open casket as dental technicians are not cheap these days". I know what you're thinking: the soda companies would never use such a slogan. It's too lengthy.

Either way, this company has successfully convinced the population that a liquid that is good for neutralising pain from insect stings, cleaning bugs from windscreens, rust removal, deodorising pets, and stripping lime build-up in toilets is something that we should all drink.

WHAT IS IT?

From the Wikipedia page on "Soft drink":

...typically contains carbonated water, a sweetener, and a natural or artificial flavouring. The sweetener may be sugar, high-fructose corn syrup, fruit juice, sugar substitutes (in the case of diet drinks), or some combination of these. Soft drinks may also contain caffeine, colourings, preservatives, and other ingredients . . . (other names are) . . . carbonated beverage, coke, fizzy drink, cool drink, cold drink, lolly water, pop, seltzer, soda, soda pop, tonic, and mineral.

Other categories of bottled drinks at the consumption gallows are bottled fruit juice, energy or sports drinks, flavoured milks, and sweetened teas and coffees. Finally, and this is pushing it but I shall explain, bottled water, mineral, and spring water. Ouch!

Bottled vegetable juice is the only bottled drink, provided it is freshly squeezed or processed, that remains on the menu.

HOW MUCH DO WE CONSUME AND WHY?

The amount of bottled drinks that we are ploughing through is cause for considerable concern given that we get most of the added sugar, 40% in an average American diet, from sweetened beverages (soft drinks, sports drinks, and 'fruit' juice). As for bottled water, ConvergEx Group Chief Market Strategist Nick Colastells says:

The [bottled water] industry grossed a total of $11.8 billion on those 9.7 billion gallons in 2012, making bottled water about $1.22/gallon nationwide and 300x the cost of a gallon of tap water . . .. If we take into account the fact that almost 2/3 of all bottled water sales are single 16.9oz (500 mL) bottles, though, this cost is much, much higher: about $7.50 per gallon, according to the American Water Works Association. That's almost 2,000x the cost of a gallon of tap water and twice the cost of a gallon of regular gasoline.[21]

Surely this has to be the biggest con of all time, to take water, often simply tap water, bottle it, label it with a nice picture of a mountain stream, call it 'mountain spring water', sell it back to us, and add yet another plastic bottle to landfills. PepsiCo was found guilty of precisely this in 2007 when their brand Aquafina was found to be nothing but treated tap water. You don't need to dig too deeply to see that cases like these are commonplace, and yet we still buy and drink the stuff in ever-growing quantities and at ever-higher prices.

———————

Why do we continue to consume this junk, even though we know it's bad for us, and in the case of bottled water can get it for nearly free from the faucet? I use to consume it almost always out of convenience and because I was led to believe it was not safe to drink faucet water. I was led astray. Here are the main reasons.

1. **Mass marketing.** Everywhere you look and in all forms of media, you are bombarded with advertising and promotion, frequently misleading, that cleverly targets victims with the power of enormous budgets that exist to create a demand that quite simply would not be there at all without it.

2. **Selective misinformation.** Whether it's fruit juice or bottled water, selective characteristics of these beverages, and of their competitors, are used in mass public misinformation campaigns. Take the fruit juice example. Promotion of fruit juice will always focus on the word 'fruit', as it in itself may be quite good for you. Fruit is not fruit juice, however, far from it. Most fruit juice is far worse for you, but this distinction falls by the wayside in order to peddle more product. There is little mention of the added sugar or the missing fibre in fruit juice as compared to fruit. And then you have the bottled water companies actively seeking to defame tap water as

unhealthy with ludicrous claims such as that public services water is only good for washing clothes and flushing toilets.

3. **Misleading labelling.** Obscene amounts of cash are spent on manipulating public perception through labelling. Labels that inform consumers about calories or sugar content 'per serving' are classic examples. The drinks manufacturer can arbitrarily decide how many servings are in a bottle or package, and then report calories or sugar per serving, not per bottle.

   Don't forget to pay attention to what Coke or Pepsi dictate to be one serving, even though when you buy a bottle you simply drink a bottle without the need for any mathematics. 'Fruit-flavoured' is another term used that should really be read as 'Contains no fruit'. The fruit flavour is produced by chemicals that trigger the same taste sensors as certain fruits. And then there's the old favourite of 'zero calories', often found in diet soda labelling and which you should stay away from as it almost certainly indicates that sugar has not been added in favour of adding artificial sweeteners. As already outlined, this is the fast track to a myriad of miserable health conditions.

4. **Renaming harmful ingredients.** HFCS, a highly processed sweetener that also extends the shelf life of products and is cheaper than table sugar, has gotten quite a bad reputation in terms of health impacts, and rightly so. It has been linked to several metabolic diseases. The big drink manufacturers know that you know this stuff is terrible, so what do they do? They rename it, of course. HFCS is subcategorised based on its fructose content. According to the *Waking Times*:

The standard HFCS–HFCS 42 or HFCS 55 contains either 42 or 55% fructose. The new term 'fructose' is now being used when foods contain the ingredient previously called HFCS-90, which has 90% fructose. Identifying HFCS-90 as 'fructose' in the ingredients list gives food makers a green light to use statements such as 'Contains No High Fructose Corn Syrup' or 'No HFCS' on the product label, thus misleading buyers.[22]

5. **Sugar addiction.** By now you should be clear from the chapters Refined Sugar and Artificial Sweeteners and Confectionery that sugar is genuinely addictive. This fact underpins all of the above reasons and is the cornerstone of the ability of the bottled drinks manufacturers' power to increase sales.

WHY ARE BOTTLED DRINKS BAD?

I've already made it clear that I am at war with sugar. Sugar in solids, as discussed in previous chapters, is not nearly the sinister enemy that is sugar in liquids. If consuming sugar in solids is like aiding and abetting the enemy, then consuming sugar in liquids is like voluntarily walking into enemy machine gun fire with a target painted on your belly after eating a magnet the size of a can of Pepsi.

One 600ml soft drink contains fifteen teaspoons of sugar. For children, each can of soft drink consumed per day increases the risk of being obese by 60% according to the New South Wales Centre for Public Health and Nutrition.[23] Soft drinks are dangerous. The fact that they have limited nutritional value is eclipsed by the fact that they don't make you feel full, so you keep eating and drinking more of that which you crave: sugar. It's a dangerous downward spiral.

Putting bottled drinks under the microscope, we see:

1. **Teeth.** Studies documented in the peer-reviewed *General Dentistry* have found that the damage caused by the citric acid in soft drinks and energy drinks to your tooth enamel is comparable to that experienced by the methamphetamine user. Energy drinks specifically have been found to detrimentally affect the contraction of the heart.

2. **Bones.** Low bone density has been related to the consumption of colas according to a 2006 study from *The American Journal of Clinical Nutrition*.

3. **Acidity.** Soft drinks are extremely acidic. One cola would require 30 cups of pH-balanced water to neutralise it. The kidneys have to work overtime to filter out this acid residue.

4. **Dubious ingredients.** Aspartame, an artificial sweetener previously criminalised, is frequently found in soft drinks, particularly diet sodas. Other soft drinks such as Mountain Dew are made with the flame retardant brominated vegetable oil (BVOs). Granted that this will prevent your soda pop from bursting into flames, which is useful, but do you really want to be drinking flame retardant BVOs? Consuming this can cause reproductive problems, depress the nervous system, interrupt the endocrine system, and create behavioural problems (especially in children).[24]

5. **Empty fruit juice.** Even the supposedly '100% pure' fruit juice in your local supermarket is not what it seems. The fruit is extracted from actual fruit, but storage over long periods of time (up to one year) in oxygen-depleted tanks tends to remove most of the flavour. The big juice companies need to add back the flavour chemically, so the juices end up a long way from being natural.

6. **Endocrine-disrupting chemicals in bottled water.** Researchers have found endocrine-disrupting chemicals (EDCs) that seem to adversely affect development and reproduction in eighteen popular bottled waters. Endocrine disruptors interfere with the hormone system and can cause cancerous tumours, birth defects, cardiovascular disorders, metabolic disorders, and other developmental disorders.[25]

7. **Bottled water quality.** Because bottled water is usually not regulated by the same authorities as tap water, often bottled water has, in fact, been of a lower quality than tap water. A recent comparison undertaken in Cleveland, USA, found that the Fiji Water brand contained traces of arsenic, whereas the municipal water supply did not.

8. **Plastic bottle mayhem.** Aside from the fact that the plastic bottles of water bought every week in the United States alone could circle the globe five times, the bottles themselves are toxic, made from all sorts of nasties. The Pacific Institute found that it takes about 17 million barrels of oil to produce plastic for the bottled water consumed by Americans, based on 2006 consumption data.[26] The same oil is needed to fuel more than 1 million American cars and light trucks for a year.

THE CLEANSE

The consumption of bottled drinks is so ingrained in our modern lifestyles and so accessible and convenient that the idea of quitting them is difficult. As such, withdrawal does not come with a well-publicised path, and this is exactly how bottled drink manufacturers want it to stay. But it can be done, and you and your planet will be grateful in the end.

Bottled drinks are also quite affordable, but this price for your wallet does not take into account the likely increase in personal health care costs, neither does it factor in the long-term cost of environmental destruction though the sourcing, manufacturing, and waste disposal of the packaging.

The main approach taken to this week's cleanse is found in the replacements, as discussed next. To emphasise why we must get off this consumable, take a look what the folks from The Story of Stuff have put together on this topic. Their wonderfully honest and informative short film, *The Story of Bottled Water*, will get you ready to exit bottled drinks.[27]

––––––

Bottled drink replacements may not be immediately obvious, but there are many. It may take a little extra effort, but your wallet and body will appreciate it.

1. **Drink tap water.** Stop listening to the negative press about tap water. Most Western municipal water supplies

are perfectly healthy and often healthier than some bottled waters. If you're a bit unsure about this, add a water purifying filter to your faucet. I live in Indonesia, where I can confirm that the tap water in large doses can make a person ill. I use a local water filter designed for tap water; it's that easy. I then reuse old wine bottles and the like, filling them with filtered tap water and refrigerating because I like cold water. You can also buy a reusable water bottle you can fill from the tap and take it with you when you are on the move.

2. **Eat and drink fruit.** Knowing now that you are most likely getting minimal if any benefit from bottled fruit juices, give them up and simply eat fruit, getting all the goodness of fruit and some added fibre, which will help keep your blood sugar levels stable. If you simply must drink your fruit, then use a food processor that does not remove all the pulp from the output.

3. **Vegetable juice.** Made using a food processor or bought freshly made, vegetable juices offer a quick, low-calorie way to get all the benefits of vegetables but with much less natural sugar than fruit juices. If you need to sweeten them, use natural sweeteners or even add some fruit. Experiment with combinations of any number of vegetables and fruit. My favourites are carrot, spinach, beetroot, avocado, celery, ginger, apple, pear, and mint.

4. **Flavoured tap water.** This is a good way to ween oneself off energy drinks for the hard-core addicts. You can start with your purchased energy drink, but start diluting it with tap water, more with each bottle, until there is hardly any purchased energy drink in the concoction. Then make the switch to flavoured tap water by just adding slices of your favourite fruit and vegetables (e.g.,

oranges, lemons, limes, watermelon, cucumber, mint) to the cold tap water in you fridge. Also try adding small amounts of essential oils such as peppermint, lemon, and orange. Even add cinnamon sticks if you fancy. You can also make ice cubes from a blended mix of water and your favourite fruits.

5. **Home-brewed ice tea.** Stop purchasing bottled ice tea, which is both black tea and all too often is loaded with sugar. Brew your own herbal or green tea at home and then refrigerate and add fruit as you like. Compared to black tea, green tea is high in antioxidants, and may help reduce the risk of several types of cancer, heart disease, hypertension, kidney stones, and cavities.

6. **Homemade pop.** If you struggle to quit soft drinks, make a one-off purchase of a water carbonator such as Soda Stream. Then just bubble tap water through it and add lemons or limes and a small amount of natural sweetener such as Stevia. You only need a minuscule amount of Stevia; otherwise, it becomes overpowering, and hey, presto! Homemade soda.

———————

Following this replacement plan will have a huge impact on your financial resources and your health. I didn't drink soda, but I was a bottled water fiend, particularly since I moved to a country where the town water is not recommended for drinking. I'm talking about at least three large purchased bottles of water a day. With my water purifier and used wine bottles, I now buy zero bottled water and zero bottled anything (except wine . . . oops).

I also am happy not to see my rubbish bin filled with plastic bottles that will contaminate some land or water somewhere. Annually, this keeps around 1,000 bottles out of the system each year. And I will no longer be at the mercy of the huge, multinational bottled drink manufacturers. These companies have no regard for your health or the health of the planet, so turn your back and walk away; you don't need them.

ACTIONS

•Watch *The Story of Bottled Water*
http://storyofstuff.org/movies/story-of-bottled-water.

•Read the labels on bottled drinks to find the truth.

•Familiarise yourself with what these drinks are and stock up on replacements.

•Free yourself from the grip of the bottled drink multinationals.

•Smile and bare your gnashers because you can.

MENU

Do Drink	Drink in Moderation	Drink If You Must	Do Not Drink
Tap and filtered tap water Vegetable juice, homemade pop, iced tea, and flavoured water	Fresh fruit juice with the pulp		Any other drink in a bottle, carton, or can

WEEK 5 - COFFEE

Coffee leads men to trifle away their time, scald their chops, and spend their money, all for a little base, black, thick, nasty, bitter, stinking nauseous puddle water.

—The Women's Petition against Coffee, 1674.

————

The coffee bean, named after the Kaffa region in Ethiopia where it was supposedly discovered in the eleventh century, has faced quite a bit of resistance in some cultures over the years. It has been blamed for fuelling riots and spawning seditious speech and Satan worship, to name a few. In Constantinople in 1623, laws were instituted to punish those in possession of coffee with a beating. Repeat offenders were quite rightly sewn into leather sacks and tossed into the river. If only those guys had had this book back then.

In today's caffeine-soaked world, I suspect we are safe from these types of accusations, but that is not to say that coffee is going to escape the Consumption Cleanse. When I see myself consuming around five double espressos daily and struggling to sleep for more than a few hours nightly, I see enough motivation to make a case for the end of coffee.

It may well be that there is quite a long list of health benefits from moderate coffee use, but the negative impacts on me and the earth, as outlined below, bear a weight heavier than a sack full of caffeine-loaded corpses.

WHAT IS COFFEE?

Coffee is a brewed beverage made from dried, roasted, and then ground coffee beans. Coffee beans are the seeds of berries from the coffea plant, found natively in Africa and some islands in South East Asia and now cultivated in over seventy countries. There are really only two types of commercially produced coffee beans: Arabica, the more highly regarded and common (70% of all coffee grown) bean, and Robusta, considered to be less flavourful, hardier, and cheaper. Robusta is typically found in instant coffee and usually has a higher caffeine content.

Decaffeinated coffee is made by mixing normal coffee with a solvent that dissolves away most, but not all of the caffeine. Why anyone would drink this substance is a mystery to me. It's like having sex without the sex. As decaffeinated coffee still contains some caffeine, it too will be eliminated from the diet.

Iced Coffee also gets removed this week, as does any other variation of coffee such as Affogato, Americano, bicerin, breve, cafébombón, café au lait, caffécorretto, cafécrema, caffélatte, caffémacchiato, café mélange, coffee milk, café mocha, caphesuada,cappuccino, carajillo, cortado, cubanespresso, espresso, eiskaffee, the flat white, frappuccino, galaogreekfrappé coffee, Indian filter coffee, instant coffee, Irish coffee, coffee liqueur, kopiluwak, Kopi Tubruk, Turkish coffee, Vienna coffee, and yuanyang, to name a few.

How Much Do We Consume and Why?

The world's population of caffeine addicts consumes 500 billion cups of coffee per year. I used to contribute just under 2,000 of those. Scandinavians consume the most coffee per capita in the world, with Finland taking the top position at four cups per day. Keep in mind that number includes children and other folks that don't indulge, so the number of cups per coffee drinker would be higher. In terms of total consumption by country, the United States consumes the most.

Coffee is the world's most sought-after commodity after oil, worth between $60–100 billion annually, depending on how you measure it. (Sources vary.[28]) Most of the associated revenue ends up in the hands of only four major conglomerates: Nestlé, Philip Morris, Procter & Gamble, and Sara Lee, which wrestle 60% of US sales.

Less than 10% of global earnings ends up in the hands of the almost 25 million coffee farmers who depend on it for their livelihood. Developing nations account for 90% of all coffee production.

These statistics hopefully highlight the sorry state of the distribution of wealth generated by coffee. Fair Trade coffee, which gives farmers a fairer go and is kinder on the environment, only accounts for 2% of global supply. So, by and large, the coffee industry is not one that I am too excited about supporting.

———————

Let's not muck around here. We consume coffee because it gives us a boost, both real and perceived, and it is quite addictive. I say 'perceived' based on my own experience when I realised that the supposed energy boost is actually overshadowed by a psychosomatic stimulus. Coffee takes about fifteen to twenty minutes to enter the bloodstream and is completely absorbed by about minute forty-five.[29] My experience was, however, that immediately after I had downed one of my five daily double espressos, I was energised and motivated. This tells me that it is the ritual and the anticipation of the actual kick that would get me moving. This comes into play when I talk about quitting and replacements.

Other reasons for consuming coffee vary. Some enjoy the art of brewing itself; others philosophise about the process and the way to imbibe it. The way it is consumed, where it is consumed, and what type is consumed are all intertwined with social and cultural background. Inversely, your social, community, and cultural rituals will often dictate this behaviour.

I can't deny that coffee has is place in lubricating our social fabric and enabling human connection, but this can be achieved with many of its alternatives as well. On the basis of its negative impacts discussed below and considering that coffee has so many good alternatives, I took it out of my diet.

WHY IS COFFEE BAD?

Caffeine is the most widely used psychoactive drug in the world. It has been found in more than sixty plants species, and dietary sources include coffee, tea, cocoa beverages, chocolate, and some soft drinks. The impacts of coffee on your health are varied and controversial. The effects on the planet are not. They are decidedly negative.

For myself, the major detectable personal impact was that coffee supported my insomnia in a massive way. I had tried numerous sleep remedies from pharmaceutical to natural remedies and from hypnotism and meditation to shamanic ceremonies involving the poisonous excretion from the sweat glands of the Amazonian Kambo frog. The only remedy that made a measurable difference was cutting out coffee. I still had to work on my sleep habits after quitting (which is another story), but since I eliminated coffee, I have been sleeping for most of the night. In addition to not sleeping, I was shedding way too many shekels for no reason.

Since cessation, I have had one single espresso, and its effects on me were huge. I broke out into a sweat, was visibly shaking, could feel my heart pumping like it wanted to escape my chest cavity, and generally felt nervous and jittery. This reaction told me that the immunity I had built up previously masked the drug's true effects.

That was my personal experience but depending on who you ask or what you read, coffee is either a super-healthy tonic or incredibly harmful.

1. **The good.** Coffee contains small amounts of vitamins and minerals, is high in antioxidants, and is linked to a reduced risk of some diseases. Caffeine, its main active compound, can cause a short-term boost in energy levels, brain function, metabolic rate, and exercise performance. Several studies show that coffee drinkers have a much lower risk of dementia, Alzheimer's disease[30], and Parkinson's disease[31] in old age. Several

sources report an association between coffee drinking and reduced risks of some cancers and cardiovascular diseases.

2. **The bad.** According to a 2005 *Advances in Psychiatric Treatment* report, "Excessive caffeine ingestion leads to symptoms that overlap with those of many psychiatric disorders. Caffeine is implicated in the exacerbation of anxiety and sleep disorders, and people with eating disorders often misuse it".[32]

The impact of the high levels of caffeine in coffee on sleep is key here.[33] Lack of sleep is behind a multitude of physical ailments. If coffee causes lack of sleep, then it is also the underlying cause of those ailments. When sleep deprivation occurs, we get irritable and moody and experience fatigue and headaches. With continued sleep deprivation the metabolism slows down, leading possibly to weight gain and diabetes, increased blood pressure, heart rhythm irregularities, poor memory, depression, and an increased susceptibility to health problems in general. Sleep disruption will vary from person to person, and those involved in excessive consumption are more likely to suffer from these symptoms. Still keen on your daily cup of Joe?

3. **The ugly.** Many folks don't like the idea of depending on an addictive drug to function, me included. But getting off coffee may not be a pleasant experience if not planned out and handled properly. It can come with some serious withdrawal symptoms. I know that I experienced mild headaches for the first couple of days and some tiredness and irritability.

However, this was only for the first couple of days. After that I found I had generally higher levels of energy that were more consistent throughout the day. I should note that withdrawal symptoms have been found to be stronger in heavy caffeine users.[34]

4. **The uglier**. Aside from my main personal reason for eliminating coffee from my diet—lack of sleep—there are some hefty planetary considerations that really put the nail in coffee's coffin for me.

Historically, coffee was cultivated at altitudes in tropical and subtropical climes under existing forest canopies. It was often cultivated with other plant species in integrated ecosystems that supported not only those native and farmed plants but also many animals and insects that used the forest canopy as their habitat. The canopy and the integrated approach prevented topsoil erosion, and there was no need for chemical fertilisers. The ecosystem was in equilibrium. However, due to recent increased demand, this equilibrium has been falling apart as the supply-and-demand discrepancy has seen the introduction of 'mono-culture farming' and 'sun cultivation' techniques. These have caused the native forest to be slashed and burned and the single crop of coffee planted in rows without a canopy, plantation style. This, together with modern day chemical fertilisers, spells higher yields for now. But these techniques applied to the delicate ecosystems where most coffee is grown will lead to carnage.

a. **Deforestation.** Traditional farmers have been encouraged to drop their sustainable ways in favour of sun cultivation. In Central America alone 2.5 million acres of forest has been slashed for this purpose. The World Wildlife Fund says that of the 50 countries with the highest deforestation rates from 1990 to 1995, thirty-seven were coffee producers.[35]

b. **Water pollution.** Coffee processing plants discharge organic pollutants into rivers and waterways. The runoff from intensive chemical fertilisers causes eutrophication (growth of algae (algal bloom) and other aquatic plants), which eventually causes overcrowding. Aquatic plants and animals then starve for sunlight, space, and oxygen.

c. **Waste.** Vast amounts of waste are produced in coffee processing. During six months in 1988, 547,000 tonnes of Central American coffee produced 1.1 million tonnes of pulp waste, which contaminated 110,000 cubic metres of water every day.

d. **Soil quality**. As sun cultivation necessitates the removal of the forest canopy, soil erosion is massively accelerated.

I don't know about you, but the picture painted here, of which I previously had no knowledge, was sufficiently grim to vindicate my decision to exit coffee consumption.

THE CLEANSE

Armed with the information above and prepared for quitting coffee with the action plan below, so you know what to expect, will give you a solid chance of success with this week's unnecessary consumable.

This plan of attack came from numerous sources. Executing it resulted in great success. After several weeks had passed and aside from one 'blowout' that left me feeling terrible and certainly drove home my reasons for cessation, I was coffee free and very much enjoying the alternatives. Here's the plan:

1. **Admission.** Like quitting any addiction, admission is step one. I was a full-fledged junky and so found it quite simple to admit that I was addicted to coffee and caffeine.

2. **Mindset.** Get your head full of all the ill effects of coffee and, more important, all of the positive things to come from freeing yourself from it, both personally and planetarily.

3. **Replacements.** Make sure you have stocked up on the replacements you plan to use and all withdrawal aids you might want are on hand. Two withdrawal aids that seem to get a good rap are red ginseng and magnesium oil. I did not feel the need for these, but if you have concerns about the scale of withdrawal symptoms or simply want to bolster your efforts, get some. Red ginseng (tinctures more so than pills) reportedly gives you an energy boost and a general feeling of well-being while supporting adrenal gland recovery from the damage caffeine has

done. Magnesium oil relieves stress and tension and promotes relaxation and proper digestion. Topical application may sting a little to start with, so avoid sensitive areas, unless you're into that sort of thing.

4. **Withdrawal aids.** On the morning of Liberation Day, if you are choosing to use withdrawal symptom aids, as soon as you wake up take your red ginseng, or apply magnesium oil after your shower. These two products should only be used for the first week of this process. Long-term use is not on the radar here.

5. **First hit.** Around the time you would normally have your first dose of coffee, or ideally slightly before, prepare your chosen replacement instead and enjoy it. Remembering the psychosomatic effect that I experienced with coffee, I now wake up and have a half a shot of coconut oil, and I have trained my brain to believe that this shot is my kick-start. I doubt it has any energising properties. It has many other wonderful benefits, but the point is that my morning ritual has not changed; only the liquid in it has changed. I let myself believe that this is the trigger for action.

6. **Breakfast.** Have a healthy breakfast so that you feel great to start the day, reinforcing that what you are doing this week feels good and is good for you.

7. **Daily.** Consume your replacement beverage at the same times or slightly before when you would otherwise take a coffee. If your replacement is green tea or any other that contains caffeine, have a second caffeine-free replacement on hand as there is no point replacing twelve coffees a day with twelve green teas a day. You won't rid yourself of caffeine that way. Perhaps mix in alternating peppermint teas.

8. **Water.** Drink plenty of water. Water will help flush out toxins and assist in reducing withdrawal headaches.

9. **Caffeine.** Ideally, at least for the first week, minimise your consumption of replacements with caffeine so that you do actually completely rid yourself of caffeine. You need a minimum of one week of freedom from caffeine in all its forms to start breaking the addiction.

Once you've given it up, you'll notice your general feeling of well-being throughout the day will improve and stabilise. Instead of my previous five double espressos each day, I now have one coconut oil half-shot and numerous teas, mostly herbal but sometimes green tea, throughout the day. I chop and change regularly, constantly experimenting (currently with fresh organic ginger), giving me the benefit of not only what I put in my tea, but the additional water I am consuming with each glass.

———————

For this week the replacements really are endless and are mostly centred on the different types of tea you can drink. Here are a few that will get you started:

1. **Organic green tea.** My personal favourite is so popular it now comes pre-packaged in a huge range of blends. I prefer a pot brewed with just the naked leaves. It's my new ritual. It does contain small amounts of caffeine, but there are decaffeinated versions. The 'decaf' version is not produced in the same way as decaf coffee and does not

use solvents. Green tea is renowned for its high levels of antioxidants and other compounds beneficial for our health.

2. **Teeccino.** This one is for those who love the taste of coffee. Its ingredients include carob, barley, and chicory root. It could be good for digestive health, and it may also have an alkalising effect on your body.[36] It comes in loads of different flavours and is brewed in all the same ways as coffee.

3. **Peppermint tea.** Although it has no caffeine it does have quite an invigorating effect. This is a good option if you need a bit of get-up-and-go in the morning without the shakes when you are coming off coffee. It also has some solid digestive benefits.

4. **Yerba mate.** You can drink this instead of coffee, but I don't recommend it in the first week because it contains quite a lot of caffeine. After you are clean of caffeine, drinking this beverage will give you a similar buzz to that of coffee. It is made from naturally caffeinated leaves of the South American holly tree and is packed with nutrients. In Argentina, where it is widely consumed, it is known to not have the same heavy crash that coffee brings. Drink it in a traditional yerba mate infuser while riding a horse, and you'll feel just like the rugged gauchos of the Argentine Pampas.

5. **Ginger tea.** Another favourite of mine, ginger tea can be purchased or made fresh. I simply boil a pot of water and chew up about an inch of ginger root and spit it out into the boiled water. It sounds a little primitive, but I find that chewing instead of chopping releases the most flavour into the brew. Don't worry about the saliva; it comes from your mouth, and it's simply going back into your mouth.

Ginger tea is energising and has traditionally been used to settle stomach problems such as bloating and flatulence.

6. **Home-brewed concoctions**. Strictly speaking, I can't call these teas because they contain no tea, but who's checking? You can add all sorts of weird and wonderful things to boiling water, so experiment. I've found my favourite home brews involve different combinations of cinnamon sticks, cloves, mint leaves, ginger root, garlic cloves, lemons, limes, and lemon grass. For sweetener I usually use honey or cinnamon powder.

The list can go on, and it's up to your individual taste and keenness to experiment. Simply preparing coffee seems quite boring to me now. I am constantly surprised by the 'tea' flavours I create, and if you do need a kick, there are options above that will give you that.

————

Drinking coffee does not cross my mind at all anymore. When I first stopped, I did have a couple days with mild intermittent headaches but no other withdrawal symptoms. After that, the first thing I noticed was how much calmer I felt both mentally and physically. And at last I could sleep.

I know that I am getting many more health benefits from the ingredients in my home-brewed concoctions than from drinking coffee, and I feel a sense of righteousness knowing that I am not contributing to the vast scale of deforestation and other calamitous environmental harm caused by coffee cultivation.

ACTIONS

• Ensure you have coffee replacements on hand and have revised the quit plan.

• Quit drinking coffee on Liberation Day.

• Save yourself and the planet in the process.

MENU

Do Drink	Drink in Moderation	Drink If You Must	Do Not Drink
All non-caffeinated teas Teeccino	Moderate yerba mate and green and other caffeinated teas for the first two weeks	No more than two cups of 'fair trade' coffee	Regular coffee, including iced and decaffeinated

WEEK 6– LAND-BASED ANIMALS

"Now I can look at you in peace; I don't eat you anymore."

—Franz Kafka

"By eating meat, we share the responsibility of climate change, the destruction of our forests, and the poisoning of our air and water. The simple act of becoming a vegetarian will make a difference in the health of our planet."

—Thich Nhat Hanh, The World We Have: A Buddhist Approach to Peace and Ecology

———————

Many moons ago I was a pescetarian. For five years I ate no animals except for those from the sea. I had been eating animals again up until I started researching for this chapter and started living with two animal liberationists. The break that I gave animals in those earlier five years was for different reasons from those I give now. Back then my efforts were largely a social, acceptance-based manoeuvre that made me feel good about myself. I was the focus.

These last few months, however, have changed me permanently on the very big topic of eating other beings that have the ability to feel things such as physical and emotional pain. This time, I can say that I won't ever eat land-based animals again. Before you switch off thinking I'm going to bark on about animal cruelty, wait. It is and it isn't about that. It does concern animal and environmental welfare and your health, but I was already aware of this to some degree. For me now it is more about a maturing, an awakening, and certainly about the act of facing the truth about what I am eating. It is about living with reality. I look back to not long ago and ask myself how I was able to live such a fantastical duality, how I was able to ignore the ugly fact of what was sitting on my dinner plate.

I must warn you that this is the most serious chapter of all. I know that doesn't sound like fun, and it might not be fun to read. But I challenge you to take it in—not just to read the words but to take the meaning in wholly. If it affects you like it did me, it will have an enormous impact on your life, your growth as a human, and your impact on other living creatures. Once I was armed with my research on this topic and sat myself down face-to-face with the truth, I found this category the easiest of all to remove from my life.

WHAT ARE LAND-BASED ANIMALS?

This chapter concerns land-based animals only. Animals of the sea are discussed in a later chapter. Yes, I know, what about ducks? I honestly don't know what to do about ducks. On the hit list are all animals from where you might get red, pink, and white animal flesh. It also includes all processed meat—

including bacon. Smoked, cured, and salted animal flesh is also the subject here.

You may notice that I am generally not referring to animals as 'meat'. I don't refer to my pet dog as meat, bones, some hair, organs, and a painful bark. I refer to her affectionately as Wolfie the dog, or sternly as Wolfington Stanley if she is caught 'gardening'. The planned commoditisation of animal flesh as 'meat' has bought us to this point by design. It helps us disassociate the 'meat' on our plate from the pig, baby cow, or battery hen from whence it came. So, I call animals 'animals'.

How Much Do We Consume and Why?

The amount of animal flesh we eat is skyrocketing. Our current economic model of competitive pricing combined with massively increased demand from a quickly increasing middle class in China, India, and other developing countries has led to the factory farming abomination. Factory farming economies of scale result in cheaper prices through lower costs per animal. But 'cost' does not include the environmental cost, the increased cost of treating related human health issues, or the sadistic cost to the animal itself. I don't know how to measure this last, but ignoring it means animal flesh is cheaper than it would otherwise be and more of it is consumed.

In the second half of the 1900s, global meat consumption increased fivefold, passing from 45 million tonnes of meat consumed in 1950 to the current 250 million tonnes. This is set to double by 2050.[37]

The numbers of animals slaughtered every year is insane. Fifty-eight billion chickens are slaughtered annually, 11 billion in China and 9 billion in the United States. There are also 1,383 million pigs, 517 million sheep, 430 million goats, and 296 million cows slaughtered yearly.[38] These numbers are frightening.

————

I consider that I have had a typical omnivorous upbringing. 'Meat and three Veg' was the staple on the dinner plate when I was a kid. Questioning why we ate meat, just like why we ate breakfast cereal would have been absurd. Cereal was in aisle 4; meat was in the cold section on aisle 11. It was all just food right? Well, by the time it gets to the supermarket it is no longer yearling calf, it is veal. This is true, and it is on that premise that the main reason we eat meat arises - blocked empathy.

We humans are generally empathetic. How is it that we can hear about cases of animal cruelty such as in the endless factory farming stories or see images and video or even the reality of it, agree that it is inhumane, and then later that day grab a hamburger for lunch? That's what I might have done. My favourite sandwich was a BLT, bacon lettuce and tomato. There is no mention of our fellow earthly animals in our foods. I didn't grab a sandwich with a slice of the arse of a pig that lived in a cell all of its life that was so small it slept standing up, did I?

Science has shown that our species has eaten other animals all throughout our evolution. That is one reason folks say that eating other animals is okay. But evolution itself is why we probably wouldn't if it weren't for certain market forces. You see, with evolution came greater intelligence and empathy.

Market forces, namely the profit motive within the meat industry, know all too well about humans' capacity for empathy. This is why mountains are moved to ensure that the disconnect between 'meat' and the animal it came from remains intact. As a kid, do you think I would have eaten veal, if the label correctly said "Baby cow stolen from its mother one day after birth, fattened in a cell, and slaughtered on its turning four months old?"[39] Of course not. The meat industry for generations has worked hard on secrecy and disassociation to ensure our empathy does not kick in and to ensure they can keep selling 'meat'. And they have done a great job.

I believe that if our empathy were to have free reign, and we were forced to meet our meat before we ate it, we wouldn't eat a great deal of it, if any. But this is only scratching the surface. I am only talking about associating the animal with the food. But the shocking reality about what is hidden from the consumer is not just the animal but the abhorrent process by which animals are raised, fattened, prepared, butchered, and sold. This applies mainly to but not only in factory farming operations. If we were all forced to acknowledge and even SEE this, we would run a mile from eating animals. I'll talk more about this later, but you can take a look at this in an eye-opening documentary called "Farm to Fridge - The Truth behind Meat Production"[40] to warm you up. I'm not here to shock, but we need to face the truth. If you can watch this reality and still feel okay about eating animals, I'd be surprised, but so be it.

The second big reason we eat animal flesh is to get protein into our diet. Protein is needed but it does not have to come from land animals. Other good sources are fish, vegetables, beans, some grains, and seeds. Proteins found in these sources are generally low in fat, whereas land animal sources are often high in saturated fats. The fact that you need animal flesh in your diet is untrue. Moreover, the recommended intake of protein is 40g per day. Animal eaters average way more than that at 80g per day, even vegetarians average around 70g.[41] It's lack of fibre that causes more health issues, and there's not a great deal of fibre in a sausage. A bean sprout or a flax seed however…

The final big reason I have used and I hear many others use is that meat tastes good. Yes it does. But this alone is no reason to eat it. I suspect that my 'Wolfie' would taste good too, particularly if I loaded her up with all the crap that we put into cows these days to maximise yield and taste. But I don't eat her. I haven't eaten any dogs intentionally for that matter. Why? Because I have pet dogs, and I empathise with them. When you meet your meat and understand their miserable lives, made so by human demand, you will empathise with those animals too and the taste will be irrelevant as it should be.

Why Is Eating Land-Based Animals Bad?

There are three areas I will cover here: animal cruelty, the impact of livestock farming on the ecosystem, and the impact of eating animals on your health.

I had considered myself fairly well versed on the topic of animal cruelty in meat production, but I found I was quite wrong. Day after day of investigating stories of impossible cruelty, even those I had thought were fiction or at least exaggerated, turned out to be true. It was a highly depressing time for me, particularly in knowing my own eating choices were part of it. Most of the acts and indeed some standards in the industry have come about in the name of efficiency to cut costs and maximise yield and profit. You'd never think I was talking about intelligent beings, would you? Imagine talking about a human like that. Actually, in some workplace environments we do. Oops. At least we're not eating each other yet.

As mentioned earlier, the manner in which our demand for animal flesh has these beings raised, fattened, butchered, prepared, and sold is appalling. The meat industry knows this, and that is why you don't see or read about it in your everyday lives, particularly about what goes on in factory farming operations. If you did, the animal flesh industry would rot away into insignificance.

Factory farming is the practice of raising usually thousands of animals in close confinement and high density with the purpose of producing meat, eggs, and dairy products in the fastest, most efficient, and cheapest way possible for human consumption. Note that I'm not including the welfare of the animals or the safety of the food produced when I say this. Common sense dictates that for food to nourish the body, it itself needs to have been nourished and well cared for, yet the gruesome holocaust for these animals is commonplace. This type of treatment is completely unnecessary, as any small farmer can tell you. Chilling examples from our world's factory farms include:

1. **Raised.** In some Western countries, calves are routinely raised for veal, after being taken from their mothers only days after birth. They are confined in individual crates too narrow for them even to turn around, they're virtually immobilised for their entire sixteen-week lives.[42]

2. **Fattened.** Growth hormones, genetic engineering, and specific breeding programs are used to create more consistently desirable animal anatomies and to stimulate growth. This potent chemical cocktail fattens only the animal parts that consumers pay most for. The animal exists solely for us to eat it.

3. **Prepared.** The miserable lives of chickens raised for meat and eggs ends at the slaughterhouse. The process of capturing them and putting them into crates is so rough-and-tumble that broken bones are common. Once at the slaughterhouse, the birds are hung upside down in shackles further injuring their legs. Machines then cut their throats before they are immersed in scalding-hot water to remove their feathers. They are often conscious throughout the entire process. They are often not stunned before their throats are cut.

4. **Butchered.** A cow can live up to twenty-five years. Dairy cows usually meet their ends at beef slaughterhouses at just five years of age, when their milk production has slowed, or when they are too crippled or ill to continue in the industry.

5. **Sold.** Millions of Australian sheep and cattle suffer unnecessarily during live export because of the almost unbearable conditions on board the ship. In suffocating conditions, they are forced to stand and sleep in their own excrement for excruciatingly long periods of time before arriving at their destination, often dead. Those not dead on arrival, if it is a Halal destination, will suffer a fully conscious slaughter, condemned to a painful and prolonged death.

You don't have to dig very deeply to see countless standard practises that are utterly inhumane. I have not included some of the most gruesome practises I came across here, as I did not want to lose your readership.

The process of raising livestock for food has a massively negative effect on our ecosystem. It's vital that you watch a documentary called *Cowspiracy: The Sustainability Secret*.[43] It sheds light on the modern-day meat industry and its relation to climate change as well as its detrimental effect on the Earth's environment. Remember, I challenge you to follow this chapter closely, to really process what I'm saying, and to be in touch with the reality. Heads do not belong in the sand. Environmental issues around raising livestock include:

1. **Inefficient land use**. The land use required to support livestock is massive, not so much for the animals themselves (In factory farming a sow will take up no more land than the size of its shadow.), but in the production and acquisition of feed and water. Seventy per cent of US grain production is used to feed farm animals. The grains and soybeans fed to animals to produce the amount of meat consumed by the average American in one year could feed seven people for the same period.[44]

2. **Inefficient energy use.** It takes twenty-eight calories of fossil fuel to produce one calorie of protein from cows. It takes only two calories of fossil fuel to produce one calorie of protein in soybeans.

3. **Deforestation**. The production of crop feed for livestock is the leading cause globally of land clearing

and habitat loss for native animals. Of the world's arable land 33% is set aside for growing animal feed.

4. **Water use**. To produce one pound of beef it takes 1,799 gallons of water; one pound of pork takes 576 gallons of water. In comparison, the water footprint of soybeans is 216 gallons, and corn is 108 gallons.[45] *Cowspiracy* tells us that animal agriculture is responsible for 20–33% of all the fresh water consumption in the world.

5. **Greenhouse gases.** According to *Cowspiracy*, animal agriculture is responsible for 18% of greenhouse gas emissions, more than the combined exhaust from all mechanical transportation.

6. **Water pollution**. The widespread use of pesticides, herbicides, and chemical fertilisers in the production of feed crops often interferes with the reproductive systems of animals and poisons waterways.

And if all of this is still not tipping the scales, there is the effect on your health:

1. **Disease.** A vegetarian diet significantly reduces your risk of heart disease, cancer (which is also closely linked to processed meat and meats preserved by smoking, curing, or salting), osteoporosis, and kidney and gall stones.

2. **Toxic chemicals**. Factory-farmed animals contain high levels of antibiotics, growth hormones, and pesticides. Meat is not just meat anymore; it is highly contaminated with industrial poisons.

3. **Sodium nitrite.** Bacon, hot dogs, and other processed meats have a special place in the 'bad for you' world. Bacon contains forty-five calories per strip and is loaded with fat and sodium. These foods all have the preservative sodium nitrite. This carcinogen has been linked to leukaemia in children, brain tumours in infants, and other forms of cancer.

4. **Meat glue.** What the?! This is an ingredient that is added to cuts of meat from the supermarket and even in restaurants. It acts as a binder to 'glue' multiple scraps together to ultimately create one steak, chicken breast, or pork chop. Known as transglutaminase, and harvested from animal blood, it is made by the fermentation of bacteria. The gluing of many pieces of the resultant Frankenstein steak traps bacteria at the joins. So when you eat such a steak that is not fully cooked, you are exposing yourself to this bacteria, increasing your risk of contracting a food-borne illness.

5. **Carbon monoxide.** This is the practice of injecting meat with deadly carbon monoxide gas so that retailers can make old meat look presentable for weeks after it should have already gone bad. It colours meat an unnatural red even as it ages on the shelf.

6. **Fattening.** Meat eaters are three times more likely to be obese than vegetarians and nine times more likely than vegans. On average, vegans weigh ten to twenty pounds less than adult meat-eaters.[46] Vegetarian diets are also associated with higher metabolic rates than those of meat eaters.

7. **Death.** Mainly due to the facts above, animal eaters just don't live as long as vegetarians and vegans. Sarah Glynn states:

According to a study of over 70,000 people published in the journal JAMA Internal Medicine, vegetarians were 12 per cent less likely to have died during a six-year follow-up period than their meat-eating peers. Vegetarian men live to an average of 83.3 years, compared with non-vegetarian men who live to an average of 73.8 years. Vegetarian women live to an average of 85.7 years, which is 6.1 years longer than non-vegetarian women according to the Adventist Health Study-2.[47]

THE CLEANSE

I found this category by far the easiest to give up. The content I've provided above is only a summary of my research effort, and while I can't, I wish I could transplant all that I have seen and read into your mind. That would end this section. You would never eat animals again. As I am not knowledgeable in this type of mental procedure, you can simply read this chapter and watch the films listed the action items at the end. I think that should do the trick. At the risk of being repetitive, the key is to truly absorb and accept the information and what it means.

But I won't leave you high and dry with just that. I've got some other tips to help you stop eating animals:

1. **Alter your mindset.** Every time you feel like eating animals, meet your meat. By this I mean think about what it is you are eating, stop thinking veal, start thinking sixteen-week-old, helpless calf who lived its entire life in a box. This is not brainwashing, this is 'un-brainwashing'. Start getting a mindset where all animals have a right to

exist as something other than as our food. They do, don't they?

2. **Read up about factory farming.** This will surely vindicate your decision to quit eating animals. You don't have to Google for long before you are inundated with stories about the cruelty and carnage that go into making your frankfurter or producing that strip of toxic bacon. Check out *Speciesism: The Movie* while you're at it for extra food for thought. As Mark Devries says, "You'll never look at animals the same way again. Especially humans".[48]

3. **Change gradually.** Unlike some categories, you don't need to go cold turkey here, although you might want to. I sure as hell did. Gradually start replacing your animal flesh with other items, opting for high-protein foods especially. Learn a few good lentil or bean recipes and slot them into your menu. I'm a dhal fiend these days. Give me dhal over meatballs any day. Once you have the basics down, it is so versatile that your imagination is the limit.

4. **Hang out with vegetarians.** I know this sounds weird, but it is quite helpful just to get out of the habit of having 'meat' around all the time. You can garner new recipes and alternatives and reinforce your choice to give it up.

5. **Play games.** Kids mightn't be so keen on addressing animal eating. Start tricking them by using a meat substitute in pasta amply covered with sauce, and lie to them about what it is. Only after they've laid waste to their plate, tell them that it was tofu.

6. **Be prepared.** Make sure you have loads of vegetables, salads, and grains on hand. Start filling plates with these first and start serving more dishes with less or no meat as

you gradually change your ways. Enjoy learning new recipes. Have fun.

7. **Stock up on replacements.** I've listed loads of high-protein foods below that are great substitutes for animals.

8. **Think of what it all means**. Pat yourself on the back. What you are doing will be contagious. Think of what you are doing for the animals and the environment. This is evolution. This is big!

————————

Meat is essentially unnecessary in our diet. Vegetarians are careful to get enough protein because they eat other stuff instead.

1. **Iron.** Beans, lentils, kale, spinach, and soy should be in your diet to make up for the iron you are no longer getting from animals.

2. **Seeds**. Flax, hemp, sunflower, and chia seeds rank high in the protein steaks (spelling mistake intended). Add them to salads, desserts, breakfast cereals, smoothies, and yogurt.

3. **Grains.** Buckwheat and quinoa (Incan super-food) are great grains you can use to bump up your protein intake.

4. **Soya.** Soya and soya products like edamame, tofu, and tempeh have a number of applications. I drool over tempeh with barbecue sauce. Tofu is great lightly seared and added to almost any vegetable dish.

5. **Quorn and seitan**. These are so-called meats you can eat when you don't want to eat meat. Both are touted as meat substitutes, and I must say, are indeed quite meaty.

6. **Dhal**. This is by far my favourite dish. Stock up on split peas, lentils, and mung beans and become a dhal aficionado. I promise you it is the most versatile and easy-to-make healthy thing going around.

Then there's stuff you can just eat more of:

1. **Eggs.** Ideally keep your own laying chickens. You'd be surprised that this is often acceptable according to your local council. Check it out. When I was a young fellow, several of my friends in urban Brisbane, Australia kept chickens for eggs, and they had five fresh eggs every day to devour. And chickens are fun, especially for kids. If you can't or won't keep chickens, then always opt for organic, free-range eggs. The things you can do with eggs are endless, and they are loaded with protein.

2. **Fish**. Subject to the Seafood chapter, get into fish, which is high in protein. Oily fish is high in healthy omega 3s. Be warned that the fish higher up in the food chain will likely contain higher levels of mercury, as discussed in Seafood. Good options today include Atlantic salmon, herring, sardines, and mackerel. Of course, non-oily fish is good as well, provided it comes from responsibly managed fisheries.

3. **Nuts and seeds**. I may have gone too far with nuts and seeds. I use them in everything. But why not? I roast and add them to salad and vegetable dishes. They just give a

bit more texture. My favourites are almonds, sunflower seeds, cashews, walnuts, and pine nuts. Peanut butter without added sugar is also on the menu.

4. **High-protein vegetables**. Vegetables not already mentioned but high on the protein scale include spouted beans and peas, broccoli, mushrooms, artichoke, mustard greens, squash, bamboo shoots, and asparagus.

Deciding to eat vegetarian is a lifestyle choice, and it can require some work. You will be unravelling a lifetime habit of eating your fellow animals. The more you plan ahead, the easier it will be.

————————

Armed with the above tactics and replacements and 'unbrainwashed' such that the reality of a carnivorous diet is firmly with you now, your switch to a mostly plant-based diet should be achievable. It is more a process of the intellect than a physiological one. But you will see some great benefits from your actions this week. Aside from the huge environmental and animal benefits, once you switch to a mostly vegetarian diet your health will improve with reduced inflammation and lower blood cholesterol levels as well as a dramatically reduced likelihood of heart disease, some cancers, and type 2 diabetes.

Eating a mostly plant-based diet also helps us lead a more compassionate life. After all, being healthy is not just about the food we eat; it's also about our consciousness, our awareness of how our choices affect the planet and all of those with whom we share it. Three times a day, our food choices have the power to repair our broken food system and the ecosystem at large, give species a fighting chance for survival, and pave the way for a truly sustainable future. It might seem obvious, but the opposite of sustainable is unsustainable—that is, it cannot be sustained. The end of existence of some species integral to the ecosystem that has already happened at our hands will happen to us.

ACTIONS

•Watch *Farm to Fridge—The Truth Behind Meat Production*
https://www.youtube.com/watch?v=THIODWTqx5E.

Watch **Cowspiracy: The Sustainability Secret**
http://www.cowspiracy.com.

•Ensure you have meat replacements on hand and have revised the quit plan. Quit eating land-based meat on Liberation Day.

•Face your fellow animals knowing that you do not eat them.

MENU

Do Eat	Eat in Moderation	Eat If You Must	Do Not Eat
High-protein vegetables, seeds, grains, and nuts Organic, free-range eggs Tofu & tempeh and other soy products Quorn, seitan, and dhal	Seafood, subject to the Seafood chapter	Ducks, because I don't know what to make of them	All red, pink, and white animal flesh of land-based animals

WEEK 7 - WHEAT

―――――

Back in the day wheat used to be wheat. Nowadays what we call wheat is so far from the original heirloom grain of yore that we really should call it something else, perhaps 'Frankenwheat', a term coined by Dr Davis in his book, *Wheat Belly*. The oldest known variety of wheat, Einkorn, first surfaced in biblical times around the Mesopotamia neighbourhood. From this fairly nutritious, low-gluten, natural grain, bread was made by simply soaking, sprouting, and fermenting the grain and then cooking it with slow-rising yeast. We have meddled so extensively with this nutritious healthy grain, primarily in the name of yield and shelf-life, that a once-healthy food is now one of the unhealthiest. What is the point of greater yield if this is the cost? This is the essence of my argument.

Today's wheat has been hybridised over and again to force it to suit Big Ag farming systems. From this still somewhat nutritious grain, today we remove all the good bits, namely the bran and the germ, leaving only the starchy carbohydrates of the endosperm (reader giggles because I almost said 'sperm'). We don't soak, sprout, or ferment anymore, we just grind, add a load of chemicals to make up for the nutrients we took away, and then bleach and bake with quick-rising yeast. Efficiency trumps goodness. On top of that most, wheat produced contains arguably dangerous amounts of hazardous herbicides.

I have no issue with bread or pasta *per se*. They are merely the innocent victims of their own ingredients. It is wheat that rubs me the wrong way. And it's only the modern versions of it that are on my radar. You'll see that you can ditch wheat and still eat pasta, bread, and other foods that are normally made with wheat without the damaging side effects.

WHAT IS REFINED WHEAT?

Most baked stuff was already covered in the Confectionery chapter. Bread and pasta made with refined wheat are the main targets this week. Also off the shopping list are crackers, chips, pastry, flour tortillas, semolina, and bulgur.

Whole-grain wheat contains all parts of the seed and is loaded with fibre, protein, and nutrients making it satisfying and nutritious. So if you want to soften your effort here, you can eat whole-grain wheat, particularly organic varieties so as to avoid the pesticides, which I'll discuss later.

Keep in mind that whole-grain bread is still out. It is usually just a few whole grains scattered about on refined wheat bread. I'll keep whole-grain wheat off the menu for myself because of the glyphosates used in its production. I think you might find it easier as well to go hard core and say no to all wheat.

How Much Do We Consume and Why?

Approximately 700 million tons of wheat are now cultivated worldwide, making it the second-most-produced grain after maize. However, it is grown on more land area than any other commercial crop. You would think that this being the case, it would at least be something that is generally good for you. It is not.

We consume the hell out of bread because it's yummy and because we always have done so. But while we've been busy consuming it, they have been busy changing the formula. Now it is still bread on the surface, but sadly, the profit motive and chemicals have made it no longer good for us. It's time to let them know that we know that by not eating wheat-based bread. Them? They? Who are they you ask? They are the large-scale producers, operators, and growers known as Big Ag whose focus is on yield instead of maintaining a healthy and nutritious product.

Why Is Refined Wheat Bad?

The low-carb, high-carb, mega-carb, no-carb, and bi-carb approach to diet is not something this book delves into. It is not a diet book. It's a book about consumption. Everyone knows bread and pasta and other wheat-based products are high in processed carbohydrates. Whether that's good, bad, or ugly is subjective and depends on the dietary trends of the day.

Disease and death, however, are a little less subjective and really not trendy at all. Modern-day wheat grains are the cause of so many documented health problems that I'd say on a personal health level, it comes second only to sugar in terms of shocker foods.

1. **Nutrient free.** I've mentioned above that in most cases the wheat used today in bread and pasta is approaching zero-nutrition status. With the bran and the germ typically removed in wheat production, any goodness goes with them.

2. **Blood sugar spikes.** As bread is high in carbohydrates, it can cause blood sugar spikes. Even whole-wheat bread spikes blood sugar faster than many candy bars.[49] But most bread uses wheat that is so refined it gets digested very quickly. This leads to even more drastic sugar spikes, and then insulin spikes in response, and the resultant blood sugar yo-yo stimulates overeating. Even worse is that a lot of bread and bread-like foods have added sugar, making them more like bakers' confection than actual bread.

3. **Glyphosates.** This is the big one. This is the bit to pay attention to. If this weren't a problem, I'd consider still eating whole-grain wheat at least. Glyphosates, the main active ingredient in common herbicides such as Monsanto's infamous Roundup® is poison. It is promoted as a poison. It has been declared a Class 2B carcinogen by the World Health Organisation. It has been the most commonly sprayed poison on wheat crops the world over,

though that is changing. Much of Europe has acknowledged its hazardous properties and has banned it. And while the public in countries like the UK, United States, Canada, and Australia want it banned, it is still in use, despite those governments' acknowledging the health risks.

We've all seen the level of public protest against Monsanto, though perhaps not as much so the lobbying and legal wriggling and wrangling that this company has to undertake to keep its product in use.

Worse, in the United States particularly, though not exclusively, some wheat crops are drenched in this toxic poison just before harvest. Those plants not yet ripened soak up the Roundup all the way to the kernel (the bit we eat). This kills the plants, making them go to seed quicker and uniformly, resulting in an easier and higher yielding harvest. Wheat consumers undoubtedly consume small quantities of Roundup, especially when harvested this way.

Glyphosate exposure, either from your environment or in the food you eat, disrupts good gut bacteria, decimating the beneficial gut microbes and weakening the intestinal wall. This makes you susceptible not only to glyphosate's side effects, but also to other toxic chemicals you encounter. Glyphosate's impacts are slow and insidious, hitting your system over many years as your cellular system gradually becomes more inflamed. The consequences of this inflammation commonly include gastrointestinal disorders, obesity, diabetes, heart disease, depression, autism, infertility, cancer, multiple sclerosis, and Alzheimer's disease.

On this topic my favourite clip shows a Monsanto lobbyist telling a press conference that Roundup is safe to drink. But when the interviewer offers him a glass of it, he loses the plot.[50]

4. **Celiac disease and gluten intolerance.** In a report in a 2013 study published in the journal *Interdisciplinary Toxicology*,[51] clear links can be seen between Celiac disease incidence and glyphosate use on wheat crops.

5. **Autism.** A recent study found an association between gluten sensitivity and autism.[52] If you have an autistic child, you might want to steer clear of wheat, at least until more supporting research has been undertaken.

6. **GMO.** So that it can tolerate greater quantities of herbicides like glyphosates, Big Ag has invented a highly modified version of wheat, affectionately referred to as 'Frankenwheat' in *Wheat Belly*. This book is considered to be the bible of the wheat-free movement.[53] GMO wheat is creeping its way into our food systems regardless of whether it has approval to do so or not. Test crops have been found to contaminate nearby non-GMO crops. It is banned as unsafe everywhere in the world, but this may be changing with lobbying from corporate interests. See the chapter on GMOs.

7. **Azodicarbonamide (ADA).** ADA is a dough conditioner used when wheat is made into bread and pastries. It's also an industrial chemical that is used in the manufacture of yoga mats, shoe rubber, and synthetic leather! Yummy. ADA can cause respiratory problems, skin irritation, and disrupt the immune system.

8. **Preservatives.** Most modern-day bread manufacturers include a myriad of additives and preservatives in their

product to extend its shelf life. Some of these have been found to cause health issues and banned; others you'll still find in your daily bread. The Food Additives chapter delves into this in more detail. In some cases, unscrupulous companies that use these preservatives, such as Coles Australia, claim their bread is fresh. The Australian consumer watchdog, the ACCC, found that their goods had in fact been made months earlier on the other side of the world, namely, in Denmark, Germany, and Ireland, before being frozen and transported to Australia.

9. **Water pollution.** As well as the herbicide discussed above, wheat consumes large amounts of nitrates and other fertilisers. The run-off from wheat farms causes widespread water pollution.

THE CLEANSE

First you need to decide if you are going full-out in this section or if you are going to allow yourself whole-wheat grains. I encourage a blanket ban on the stuff. Seek it out in your diet and remove it. For me, the poisons and additives in this food render it inedible. The fact that it generally has no nutritional value also played a role. I'd rather get my teeth into bread and pasta that are actually doing me some good!

Start reading the labels of the packaged food you buy. That includes beer if you have not given it up. You can only drink non-wheat beers. If a product is gluten-free, it is also wheat free, but if a product is listed as wheat free, it does not mean that it is gluten-free. For example, barley and rye flour may be wheat free, but not gluten free.

The main game here can be achieved by rummaging through the replacements I discuss below and experimenting. There's so much good food out there that I was hardly noticed scrapping wheat. My latest pasta experiment is to use zucchini strands lightly cooked in a small amount of coconut oil as pasta. It rocks!

———————

There are loads of options to choose from when replacing wheat in your diet. You can make the most of what you can make with wheat with other grains. But beyond that and better, you can use vegetables as well, such as my zucchini pasta. I subscribe to quite a few vegetarian and vegan websites that regularly send out gluten-free recipes. Do the same. These websites are in the Actions section at the end of this chapter.

So, what can you use for flour?

1. **Buckwheat.** Buckwheat contains no gluten and is rich in protein. I was surprised to learn it is actually a member of the rhubarb family. The seeds can be ground into a flour to make bread, pasta, and pastries with a slightly nutty taste.

2. **Almond meal.** This is made by grinding blanched (skin removed) almonds. It's high in fibre and healthy fats. I've mixed this with other non-wheat flours as it adds moisture, flavour, texture, and nutritional value to gluten-free baked goods.

3. **Quinoa and amaranth.** Quinoa, lately touted as a 'super food' was a staple of the ancient Incan diet. They called it

the grain of the gods. Amaranth seeds can either be eaten whole in cereal or ground into flour for baking. Both of these are higher in protein and amino acids than wheat.

4. **Rice flour.** Also gluten free, rice flour is about 7% protein and is a good substitute for wheat flour in baking. The best rice breads are those made from brown rice flour.

And for some more tasty breads:

1. **Spelt bread.** This is a good choice if you can digest gluten. Spelt was an important staple in parts of Europe from the Bronze Age to medieval times. It now survives as a boutique crop in Central Europe and Spain. It has found a new market as health food and is not likely to be victim to Roundup poisoning and genetic modification.

2. **Rye bread.** This is darker and denser than regular bread and much higher in fibre. It doesn't cause the blood sugar spikes to the same extent as wheat bread, but it might take bit of getting used to in terms of taste.

3. **Cauliflower bread or pizza crust.** Making bread or pizza crusts with a mix of cauliflower and cheese is popular amongst the no-wheat tribe. To make it, grate an entire head of cauliflower and then cook it. Then mix the cauliflower with egg, cheese, and spices before it is flattened and baked.

And great pasta varieties:

1. **Rice and quinoa**. Not so many folks are keen on making their own pasta. But if you are dining out, look for pasta made from rice or quinoa.

2. **Vegetable pasta**. This is for those keen to experiment. My lead researcher, who happens to be my brother, put me on to this, and it's awesome. Use a potato peeler to skin a zucchini down to just before the seeds, and then splice those peeled bits down to the thinness that you prefer for your pasta. Lightly fry this in a splash of coconut oil and then remove from heat and let dry on a paper towel or something similar. Try it out with other vegetables. You are only limited by your imagination.

And if you simply must eat wheat bread, choose breads made from organic sprouted grains. Sprouting begins the enzymatic action that starts to break down the gluten. A good example is Ezekiel. It is made with several types of sprouted grains and legumes, including wheat, millet, barley, spelt, soy beans, and lentils. Just make sure that whatever option you go for does not contain hydrogenated oil, high fructose corn syrup, bleaching, enriched flour, wheat gluten, artificial flavour, sugars, or artificial sweeteners. It's easier just to use a replacement, isn't it?

————

Modern wheat should be avoided. That's it. It may have had some semblance of health to it in the past, but the wheat that people are eating today is completely different. Like many modern foods, when scientists try to improve on nature, they often get it wrong.

Because I was quitting nonsense foods each week back-to-back, I can't tell you what food category was having what effect. It's not very scientific, I admit. In any case, I continued to lose flab, and I suspect this week's category contributed to that a lot. The weight melting away was most likely due to the drop in my blood sugar. I stopped getting that bloated feeling from meals with wheat, and I don't seem to experience PFC (post-food coma).

I still see Vegemite toast and experience minor drooling. But when I think about what is in it, I ditch the toast and just scoop a thumb's worth directly from the jar, and I feel sated. I like that I don't go into bakeries anymore. They smell great from outside, but inside the gravitational odour would seduce me into purchasing not just the intended loaf of bread, but also a Neenish tart and a chocolate brownie. I don't have that exposure anymore. That weakness is stifled at the bakery door.

As I write this I can report one blowout. In an attempt to combat a hangover, I had a cheeky Mexican burrito with a flour tortilla. I can assure you that while I didn't beat myself up about it, I did feel a bit beat up after the sugar rush departed, and my hangover was only worse. Again, I accept that this is not really a scientific approach.

I don't struggle without bread in my diet. The alternatives are plenty, and restaurants are wising up. When you look at them, wheat-based bread and pasta are not something that you need to be eating, let alone poisoning yourself with.

ACTIONS

•Watch *The War on Wheat*
https://www.youtube.com/watch?v=eO3cIrNEuIc.

•Do yourself a favour and decide to replace wheat in all its forms.

•Do some research and stock up on wheat replacements.

•Subscribe to the following websites for great wheat free recipes

http://www.onegreenplanet.org

http://www.jamieoliver.com/recipes/category/special-diets/gluten-free

http://www.wheat-free.org/recipes.html

MENU

Do Eat	Eat in Moderation	Eat If You Must	Do Not Eat
Buckwheat, almond meal, quinoa, amaranth, and rice flours Spelt, rye, and cauliflower breads Pasta made from rice, quinoa, and vegetables		Organic whole-grain wheat products	Bread and pasta made with refined wheat Crackers, chips, pastry, flour tortillas, semolina, and bulgur

WEEK 8 - DEEP FRIED

"Broccoli might get stuck in your teeth, but French fries will get stuck on your ass."

—Anon

—————

The seaside town where I spent most of my thirties had a seafood shop that was famous for its deep-fried Mars bars. They even had a picture of the newspaper article that featured this odd 'seafood' in the window of their shop. Needless to say, every tourist who saw this clipping swarmed like flies on a turd to get one and eventually gagged on it. Now that I picture it, it did look remarkably like a turd. The locals knew that it was something so disgusting and ridiculously unhealthy that no amount of novelty would draw them in. A chocolate bar, coated in beer batter, deep-fried in filthy fishy oil, coated in icing sugar, and then sold by a seafood shop defies the Consumption Cleanse regulations a whopping five times! (Seafood will be discussed in a later chapter.) It is actually sweet on the first, nervous nibble. But after that it is frighteningly sickening. Everything beneath the outer sugar layer gets fused into a homogeneous orgy of dietary badness only held rigid by the bloated, fishy batter.

When something is deep fried, particularly in batter, it is typically done at a temperature higher than what the oil can withstand without changing into something toxic. This ensures a crispy, tasty outcome but also promises that what comes out of the vat is not what went in. You might call it a kind of alchemy, although I doubt alchemy can be blamed for the deep fried rat found in a California man's KFC chicken nuggets, if you choose to believe the urban legend. But who can know, stranger things have happened. Or have they?

For my money, besides the major negative health implications associated with deep frying, I want my food to resemble its form when it was alive as closely as possible, without its actually being alive. I want it to retain the nutrition it had before it was tormented in boiling hot oil.

What Is It?

Deep frying is as old as the hills. But this does not mean it is good for you; syphilis is also as old as the hills. Almost always, deep-fried food is extremely bad for you. There is a way to make deep frying a healthy option, but you won't find it applied anywhere outside your own home. There is a specific manner in which to do it that I discuss in the Cleanse section towards the end of this chapter. So, I will make it easy and include in this category everything that is deep fried, excluding that one method.

Included this week is all the obvious stuff like fast-food, deep-fried chicken parts, fish, French fries, and I suppose rats to be complete. Also consider all variants of the French fry such as potato wedges and fries made of other vegetables. Then you have all that lovely seafood done in batter, schnitzels, and anything cooked tempura style. There are all sorts of weird and wonderful faux foods that go through the hot oil at carnivals and fairs. The height of mankind's culinary evolution brings us the Dagwood Dog, the battered *sav*, the corn fritter, the deep-fried spring roll, and the dim sim.

There were some unexpected foods that I was not happy to see go because I had started eating them even more since starting this cleanse. I did an inventory of what I ate—well, what I was still permitted to eat. Sadly, I had to say goodbye to many of the tofu and tempeh varieties I was eating. I found they were deep fried, not just fried. Much Indian food gets the oil treatment such as onion bhajis along with representatives from Mexico such as the chimichanga. I also turned my back on the humble donut, falafel, and prawn chip.

Deep frying is everywhere, so be on you guard. I certainly had to start customising most meals that I ordered in restaurants. I was becoming a pain in the arse, and I wasn't even halfway through the cleanse!

WHY IS DEEP FRYING BAD?

Don't you just look at stuff in those deep fryer vats and know it shouldn't go into your body? I confess I did like to have French fries accompany my bun-less organic vegetable and tofu burger, but it turns out that deep-fried potatoes are the worst of the worst. Check out this profusion of issues with eating deep-fried food.

1. **Trans fats.** Hydrogenated or partially hydrogenated vegetables oils (Trans Fats) are commonly used in the deep fryers of restaurants the world over. Trans fats raise your cholesterol, harden your arteries, and increase the likelihood of heart disease. They contribute to inflammation in your body, insulin resistance, and Alzheimer's disease.

2. **Overheating.** To get that crispy batter effect, oil generally needs to be heated to a higher temperature than one at which it can remain stable. When oil is overheated or oil is overused, oxidation and polymerisation occur. This leaves the oil and the products cooked in it tasting rancid and packed full of free radicals and other toxic compounds.

3. **Good oils.** The smoke point of some common good oils, such as extra virgin olive oil (160°C), is typically lower than other oils. Bringing these oils up to around 180°C, the typical temperature required for deep frying, exceeds their smoke point at which the oil turns toxic.

4. **Overuse.** Most restaurants will only change their oil daily, at best. Using oil over and over again increases the breakdown and oxidation process.

5. **Cancer.** When carbohydrate-rich foods such as potatoes are deep fried, they produce acrylamide, a carcinogen associated with cancer. Check out the short clip about the danger of French fries from the folks at nutritionfacts.org.[54]

6. **Nutrition.** The deep-frying process destroys a lot of the useful vitamins and minerals in the food.

7. **Brain malfunction.** Some oils like sunflower and flaxseed oil break down and produce toxic aldehyde when heated

for long hours. Aldehyde compounds increase the risk of neural disorders.

8. **Flammable.** Of course, oil is flammable. Deep fryers are the leading cause of house fires in the United Kingdom according to the Wikipedia page on "Deep Frying".

9. **Waste oil.** Finally, deep frying produces loads of waste oil. This is often disposed of down the drain, overflowing sewer systems, sticking to pipes, and wreaking havoc in sewerage treatment systems.

THE CLEANSE

Deep-fried food in batter is only addictive to the extent that what's inside the batter is addictive. So unless you're eating deep-fried Mars bars, there is no addiction in most cases. Sugary deep-fried foods like donuts are addictive because sugar is addictive. Other than police departments around the world and their very special relationship to donuts (and I don't have a clue why that exists), I don't see a lot of addictive behaviour with deep frying.

So, in terms of how to give it up, there is no twelve-step program or anything like that. It's as simple as having good alternatives on hand.

———————

1. **Cooking style.** Eating out or at home, instead of deep-fried recipes choose the grilled, boiled, or baked options.

This would apply to a lot of fish and other seafood, for instance.

2. **French fries.** Either choose the mashed potato option or salad instead of fries. Fries are shocking. You don't need them. You might be lucky enough to stumble across pan-fried 'chips', in which case you have the green light. Certainly, at home, boil and bake or boil and pan fry on low heat using healthy oils like coconut or cold-pressed extra virgin olive oil.

3. **Home deep frying.** If you do this yourself and control the process and ingredients you might not have to bring forward your big day at the crematorium. The first thing to note is that temperature is key. Too cold and you get a soggy result; too hot and the oil breaks down and all the bad stuff above happens. So, get a good food thermometer. Deep frying works best at 176–190°C (350–375°F). Oils that have the most saturated and monounsaturated fats are the most stable when heated. You also need an oil that has a 'smoke point' high enough to give you a crispy result. Coconut oil is loaded with the right fats, and its smoke point is 177°C degrees Celsius, which   is   perfect. Set your temperature to 177°C degrees and certainly no higher than 180°C degrees as every degree above that will make the oxidation process exponentially worse. Studies have shown that even after eight hours of continuous deep frying at 180°C (365°F), this oil's quality does not deteriorate.[55] Also note that you need to keep the oil fresh.

———————

I don't eat deep fried food at all now. The home preparation method is too scientific for me, and you still have all that waste oil anyway. Get rid of it completely if you can. You'll have fewer options to deliberate over on menus. In fact, for me now, it's getting to the point where I need to bring my own food to restaurants, taking 'BYO' (Bring Your Own) to the next level.

You know when you look at this food that it's junk. It might give you some short-term taste pleasure, but it's not worth it. Don't you want to live forever? I do.

ACTIONS

•*Watch Cancer Risk from French Fries*
http://nutritionfacts.org/video/cancer-risk-from-french-fries.

•Decide to go hard core and abandon deep frying or get a food thermometer.

•Quit deep-fried food on Liberation Day.

MENU

Do Eat	Eat in Moderation	Eat If You Must	Do Not Eat
Grilled, boiled, or baked alternatives Mashed potato	Pan-fried food cooked with coconut oil	Home deep-fried food according to the instructions above	Anything deep fried (other than at home using the method prescribed above)

WEEK 9 - GMOS

"Anyone that says, 'Oh, we know that GMOs are perfectly safe,' I say is either unbelievably stupid, or deliberately lying. The reality is, we don't know. The experiments simply haven't been done, and now we have become the guinea pigs."

-- Dr David Suzuki

————————

Edible undies made from genetically modified (GM) cotton were the only skid marks of irregularity, so to speak, wiped across the pages of this chapter. This edible form of clothing posed a quandary for me of the same calibre as those damn ducks did, and still do, in the Land-based Meat chapter. You see, my focus in this chapter is on GM food. I am okay with ignoring the topic of GM clothing, but this is food disguised as clothing, or vice versa. How can I appease fans of edible undies? What do I say to those who can't stop eating them?

Well, thanks to my relentless research and hard-nosed investigative resolve, the lights all went on for me late one night. It dawned on me, folks, that if certain undies are indeed edible, they almost certainly are not going to be made from cotton.

What Are GMOs?

Almost 100% of GM crops on the market are genetically engineered with either one or both of just two GM traits: herbicide tolerance and insect resistance. These two traits account for almost all of the GM crops grown commercially over the past twenty years.

The foods that are genetically modified or contain genetically modified organisms (GMOs) vary from country to country. I have organised this category into sections on the United States, Canada, Australia, and Europe. Apologies to the other 192 countries, but it is fairly easy to identify the GM whole foods there. Processed and packaged foods, however, include so many ingredients that go by so many names that it is virtually impossible to evict GMOs from your diet altogether without being a food detective. This is particularly the case in countries such as the United States and Canada where it is not mandatory to label GMO food.

Something else to be aware of is that there is a lot of imported GM food flowing around the globe, mostly from the Americas. These are mainly found as ingredients in processed food. This is set to increase with the introduction of new global trade deals, so be aware of other countries' GMO status if you are not buying locally produced whole food.

Here is a breakdown of GM whole foods.

1. **Corn.** Corn and corn products are some of the most prominent GMO foods around. Almost all US corn and three quarters of Canadian corn is now grown from GM

seed. In Europe one strain of modified corn is approved and cultivated, but there is a growing movement away from GMO food with several EU countries now banning it. No corn grown in Australia is modified. Corn is largely included in processed foods as oils, glucose syrup, fructose and high fructose corn syrup, maltodextrin, and thickener/modified starches (additives 1410, 1412). To be safe, avoid corn and all corn products unless you know it comes from a certified organic source.

2. **Soy products.** Biotech giant Monsanto has a stranglehold on the soybean market, with approximately 90% of US soy and 80% of Canadian soy being genetically engineered to resist their herbicide Roundup. Australian soybeans are GM free, but that does not mean soy products are because they can contain imported GM ingredients. Europe imports almost all of its soy from countries that grow a GM version of it. Soy is found in tofu, vegetarian products, soybean oil, soy flour, soy lecithin (additive/emulsifier 322), soy oil, soy protein, vegetable protein, and numerous other products.

3. **Canola oil.** Canola oil, produced from rapeseed, is often described as 'vegetable oil' and is one of the most chemically altered foods available. The first canola was grown in Canada, after which it was named Canada Oil to distinguish it from non-edible rapeseed. About 90% of Canadian and US canola is genetically modified. In Australia it is only 10%, and it is banned in Europe. Be sure to check what country your canola oil comes from or just avoid it altogether.

4. **Cotton.** Almost all US, Canadian, and Australian cotton is genetically modified. In Europe it is banned. Cotton is primarily used to make cotton thread but is also used to

make cottonseed oil. This oil is often labelled as 'vegetable oil' and is commonly used for deep frying. Cottonseed meal is used in animal feed. Leftover cotton fibres, too short to use in textiles, are used in food additives E460 and E461. So, unless you get around in a burlap loincloth it's not easy to avoid GMO in clothing, though you can avoid it in your food.

5. **Sugar beets.** If an inorganic product made in North America lists "sugar" as an ingredient (not 'pure cane sugar'), then it is almost certainly a combination of sugar from both sugar cane and GM sugar beets. In Europe and Australia GM sugar beets are not grown, but they are imported.

6. **Papayas.** This one may come as a surprise. GMO papayas have been grown for consumption in Hawaii since 1999. Though they can't be sold to countries in the EU, they are welcomed with open arms in the United States, Canada, and Australia.

7. **Zucchini and yellow squash**. Closely related, these two squash varieties are modified to resist viruses and are grown on a small scale in North America only. Keep an eye on imported versions if you're in Australia and Europe.

8. **Meat and dairy.** GM corn and soy are so dominant in the United States and Canada that almost all meat and dairy comes from animals fed GM crops. In Australia and Europe this is not the case with GM animal feed limited to that which is imported and cotton meal. Additionally, US meat and dairy products may come from cows injected with GM bovine growth hormone. If you don't see labels stating No rBGH, rBST, or artificial hormones, chances are the products include them. Monsanto's rBGH, a growth

hormone likely containing genetically modified components, has been banned in twenty-seven countries including Australia, Canada and those in the EU.

HOW MUCH DO WE CONSUME AND WHY?

Corn, soy, and cotton are the main mutants of the global GMO experiment. The United States, Brazil, and Argentina are the main producers of these 'Frankenfoods' with 181 million, 104 million, and 60 million acres, respectively, under cultivation. These numbers do include minor acreages of other, less significant GM crops such as zucchini and papaya.

According to International Service for the Acquisition of Agri-Biotech Applications (ISAAA)[56] statistics, GM acreage has grown more than 100-fold from the 4.2 million acres planted in 1996 when it was first commercialised. It also states that record 448 million acres were planted in 2014 and up 15 million acres from 2013. And lastly it states that GM crops are now planted in twenty-eight countries, many of which are resource-poor, developing countries.

Throughout the ISAAA website the initial impression one gets is that GM food is doing the third world a favour. You'd be excused for interpreting that these countries are swarming behind the GM bandwagon in rabid droves. However, checking out some of the numbers in this publication and elsewhere exposes that the ISAAA has more pro-GMO bend in it than a heavily pregnant mutant corn stalk. It doesn't say that only ten countries grow almost 100% of GM crops. Neither does it highlight that the top three counties account for 77%. Based on acreage, the developing countries that have been roped into using GM crops are hobby farmers at best and reluctant participants at worst.

————

I found many examples where pro-GMO groups are touting success in developing nations. The intended impression is that of global food supply saviour, but the glossy websites and selective statistics can be easily exposed.

In 2014, Bangladesh, reportedly the twenty-eighth country to embrace GM crops, only planted thirty acres in total of an insect-resistant eggplant. While pro-GM groups carried on about this model of success, the reality was slightly more sinister. The GM eggplant was hurried though the approval process, there was no public consultation, and farmer and consumer backlash were ignored.[57] Sounds familiar, doesn't it? Surely, I mean surely there were no cash-laden handshakes involved, were there?

As it happens, the independent development policy research group UBINIG spoke to 72% of the 110–120 farmers who got suckered into this deal by their own government.[58] They reported poor yields, high chemical use, and a great deal of government interference. The report states, "According to the farmers, most of the time, the officials took care of the plants themselves as they had to show a good performance." The extent to which the government officials got involved was borderline comical. They replaced dead and dying plants, applied banned pesticides, and instructed farmers to display 'pesticide free' signs on their produce. Despite all of this, most of the farmers said it was a worthless crop, and only one of the 120 said he would use it again.

In Mexico, Sudan, and Columbia, GM corn introduction has been hammered with controversy, protests, and lawsuits. This wouldn't be happening if there were an appropriate level of public engagement. I suspect the only engagement was between corporate interests and cash-strapped governments, and we've all seen that scenario before.

In India, where Monsanto owns almost all of the cotton seed supply, a similar debacle is unfolding. Small landholder farmers are experiencing drastic crop failures over and again, but they have no choice but to use the monopoly-provided seed supply. According to Vandana Shiva, a prominent Indian-born environmentalist, approximately 250,000 Indian farmers have committed suicide due to financial stress because of failed Monsanto cotton crops and the price of their cotton seed. Ironically, many decided to drink Monsanto pesticide to do the job. I guess it's good for something. Check out *Bitter Seeds*, a 2011 documentary by American filmmaker Micha Peled.[59] The film covers biotech farming in India and the impact of GM cotton on India's farmers.

These cases highlight that despite the official line, GM crops are not necessarily being grown by choice, and they are not always grown successfully.

WHY ARE GMOS BAD?

The three main arguments floating around about GM food seem to be about labelling, whether or not it can supposedly 'feed the world', and the safety of GM foods. I'm not going to get into the labelling discussion because, for me, as long as there is a question around safety, it should be labelled. We should have the choice and the ability to decide for ourselves whether or not it is safe to eat GM food.

GM companies also try to validate their existence by claiming GM crops will help feed the world because the increased yields will stretch existing arable land to produce more food for the people who need it and for future population growth. How noble, and what nonsense.

Genetically engineered crops in general have shown no increase in yield and no decrease in pesticide use. GMOs have come about to withstand more pesticide and herbicide use, not to increase yield. Even Monsanto doesn't deny this. This notion is also supported by the Union of Concerned Scientists' 2009 report "Failure to Yield",[60] the definitive study to date on GM crops and yield.

Additionally, an International Assessment of Agricultural Knowledge, Science and Technology for Development (IAASTD) report, authored by more than 400 scientists and backed by 58 governments, said GM crop yields were highly variable; in some cases, yields even declined. They concluded that the current GMOs "have nothing to offer the goals of reducing hunger and poverty, improving nutrition, health and rural livelihoods, and facilitating social and environmental sustainability."

Indeed, much sustainable non-GM farm technology has been more successful in growing yields. If these companies were concerned about feeding people, instead of selling seeds and pesticides, they could divert the vast amount of money spent on GMOs to those safer and more reliable technologies.

And finally, what about the safety of GMOs in our food? It is still highly controversial. On the one hand, you've got government agencies and the companies that profit from its sale saying that it is safe. From my snooping around, this appears to be mostly based on short-term research carried out by parties with vested interests. On the other hand, most, if not all, independent research that I found was either not conclusive or reported negative effects. The Hindustani Times remarked:

There are over 500 research publications by scientists of indisputable integrity, who have no conflict of interest, that establish harmful effects of GMO crops to human, animal and plant health, and on the environment and biodiversity... On the other hand, virtually every paper supporting GM crops is by scientists who have a declared conflict of interest or whose credibility and integrity can be doubted. [61]

Where does the truth lie? I don't trust research carried out by folks that stand to profit from a particular outcome, and I'm not sure if you have detected this yet, but I don't trust government. I pay attention to independent, peer-reviewed research and to common sense.

Here is just a fraction of what I discovered about the risks and hazards of GMOs. Starting with the macro observations:

1. **Unknown risks.** While the many identified risks are often disputed, it is generally accepted that modified food has not been proven to be safe to eat. But what is scarier than this is the unknown risks that even the seemingly corrupt health agencies acknowledge must exist with approved food. Steven M. Druker's landmark book *Altered Genes, Twisted Truth: How the Venture to Genetically Engineer Our Food Has Subverted Science, Corrupted Government, and Systematically Deceived the Public* goes into the 1992 FDA declaration that GM food is safe to eat, unless proven otherwise.[62] This left the testing of GM food discretionary for the likes of Monsanto and Syngenta. If you want to

have bulletproof arguments about the safety of GMO foods, grab a copy of his book; it's a compelling read.

2. **Banned in many countries.** In 2015 Russia completely banned all food production using GMOs based on their independent research. China and Japan also have full bans. More than half the twenty-eight countries in the European Union, including Germany and France, have decided to ban their farmers from growing genetically modified crops. Several regions, including Northern Ireland, Scotland, and Wales, have also joined the movement. Is this not saying something?

3. **Track record.** GMO giant Monsanto has a shocking track record of producing dangerous and often deadly chemical compounds such as DDT, Agent Orange, saccharin, and bovine growth hormone. Monsanto meanwhile told us all of these were safe.

4. **Desperate to avoid labelling.** These companies know that if GMO food is labelled correctly, fewer people would buy it. The US Environmental Working Group, a nonpartisan environmental defence organisation based in Washington, DC, tells us Big Food and friends spent $101.4 million last year trying to persuade lawmakers to oppose GMO labelling. And they've gone a step further now and have almost succeeded (and possibly will have by the time this book is published) in introducing via Republican senators what critics are calling the "DARK Act" – the "Deny Americans the Right to Know Act". This act essentially prohibits US states from enacting their own legislation to label GMO food.

What about the personal health issues? Many tests involving glyphosate (a main ingredient of herbicides) have been carried out on animals with some freaky-looking beasts coming out the other side. I've seen some bizarre and sometimes massive tumours on these poor critters. Other research has shown organ damage, gastrointestinal and immune system disorders, accelerated ageing, and infertility. Human studies are less common and less conclusive but do show us how GM food leaves materials behind inside us, possibly causing long-term problems.[63] I listed twenty-two different and serious ailments in animal testing including on mammals that looked likely to be caused by GM food and low levels of the accompanying glyphosate. Here are just a couple of the shockers.

1. **Kidney damage.** *The International Journal of Environmental Research and Public Health* has linked glyphosate runoff in Sri Lanka to a glaring rise in a fatal unknown chronic kidney disease.[64]

2. **Inflamed stomach and uterus**. GM corn was fed to pigs, which resulted in gross stomach inflammations and enlarged uteri. It's important to note that pigs have a physiology similar to humans.[65]

3. **Mental and metabolic damage.** In Japan, a modified bacterium created a new kind of amino acid, which was used in protein drinks. Before they could pull the product it had caused cases of severe mental and metabolic damage to hundreds and several deaths. This was the trigger for Japan to ban GMOs.[66]

4. **Stomach lesions.** GM tomatoes were discovered to cause stomach lesions in research mammals.[67]

5. **Tumours.** GM corn fed to rats was observed to cause tumours. Interestingly, even though this research was peer reviewed and survived much critique at the time, it has since been retracted. I didn't get to the bottom of why, but I got far enough to realise that there were non-scientific forces behind it.[68]

And then there are numerous environmental issues which are not disputed.

1. **Increased herbicide use.** Since the '90s when GM crops first modified the landscape forever, glyphosate (Roundup) use has gone through the roof. This is not only bad for farmers' health but for many birds, insects, amphibians, marine ecosystems, and soil organisms. Bees, the world's pollinators, and butterflies are the most talked about non-target organisms to suffer. The mass die-off of bees was so clearly linked to pesticides that the USDA tried to put a stop to the research of the whistle blower whose report was so damning.[69]

2. **Increase of herbicide-resistant weeds.** Over time the application of herbicides on crops produces herbicide-resistant 'super weeds'. These then drive the use of more and more herbicide, and the initial advantage of herbicide-resistant crops is greatly diminished or lost altogether.

3. **Contamination of organic and conventional (non-GMO) crops.** Unintended cross-pollination affects the genetic integrity of natural crops. Once these mutant genes are out of the bag and non-target species take on the altered genetic material, there is no going back.

Nature is compromised. Also, once an organic or non-GMO farmer's crop is infected, he can no longer claim to be such, which often results in financial hardship. South Korea, which has banned the cultivation of GM crops, currently has to deal with uncontrolled GM crops popping up across the country. The concern is that these uncontrolled GM strains will disrupt local ecosystems.[70] In Australia some 800 GM crop experiments have been undertaken including GM wheat, sugar cane, grapes, pineapples, papaya, and bananas. The crops are grown in open air where they pose contamination risks to the natural environment and non-GM crops.

The bottom line is that GMOs have not been proven in any way to be safe, and most of the studies actually suggest the opposite is true. This is why many countries have banned GM crops and foods. In America, they aren't necessarily labelled, much less banned, so the majority of the populace has no idea that they are eating lab-altered DNA on a daily basis.

Seeing some of the conclusive research on animals and knowing that GM material does get left behind in human systems are enough for me. And this is on top of the actual environmental damage and the history of deceit of the GMO companies. It's not hard to join the dots and declare it's too risky for now.

THE CLEANSE

I don't think it's simply a matter of quitting GMO food. It's a matter of identifying it in the face of the massive effort to keep it hidden. You might still think that the evidence against GMOs is not a resounding 'stay the hell away from it'. You might think I'm just a painful anti-establishment naysayer who jumps on every conspiracy bandwagon that rolls through town. But you surely cannot say that the evidence is clear and GMOs are good for you and good for the planet. So why take the risk when there is no need to? The best advice and my position on this is to avoid all GMOs. The question then concerns how you can do that.

I have identified what whole foods are potential GMO candidates in the "What Are GMOs?" section. Avoid them all. In terms of wearing GMOs, such as cotton knickers, well, that's up to you, but don't eat them. I have a few pointers that I observe to help me minimise the GMOs in my food.

1. **Eat local whole food.** By far the easiest way to avoid GMOs is to avoid processed and packaged food and eat fresh, local, whole foods. You can easily find out which whole foods are GM in your country and avoid them. Processed and packaged food is a complicated beast. So many additives come from imported corn-based and soy-based GMOs. It would be nearly impossible to identify and trace them all. And there are no laws to demand such ingredients be labelled.

2. **Buy certified organic.** Even if you are eating non-GMO whole foods, you might still be chomping down

glyphosate. It is used on most non-organic crops as well. Certified organic food cannot contain GMOs and cannot have used a glyphosate herbicide. Look for labels that say "100% organic", "organic", "made with organic ingredients" and "non-GMO project" if in the United States. Yes, organic food is more expensive, but the more people demand organic food, the greater will become the supply, and the lower the price. It's economics.

3. **Avoid supermarkets.** GM ingredients are in an estimated 70% of processed food in supermarkets. It's mindboggling how many ingredients go into processed foods these days. Food should not contain ingredients; food should be the ingredients. Soy flour and soy lecithin are in almost every processed item on the shelves. Shop at local markets, organic co-ops, and even online. Better than all of these options is to grow your own food.

4. **Avoid suspect ingredients.** If you must buy processed food, then avoid ingredients that are known to contain GMOs. This will be tough; it's likely that at least some of these will be in almost everything. Ingredients like whey, xanthan gum, glutamate, hydrolysed vegetable protein, lactic acid, cellulose, citric acid, maltodextrin, and diglycerides should be avoided.

5. **Become a food detective.** Labelling of minor ingredients is compulsory only in some countries. If a supplier has a product that is organic or known to contain no GMOs, they'll often label it as such, knowing it is a more desirable product; otherwise, you need to figure it out. You can check out products and ingredients on the Internet or even an app to help you identify it. Check out GMO Checker and Label GMO apps for smartphones.

6. **Milk, meat, eggs, fish, and honey.** Ensure that these animal and animal-based products are labelled 'grass-fed' or 'organic' so that you know they were not raised on GMO feed. If not labelled, ask you butcher or producer to clarify it. Additionally, meat products may be from cows injected with GM bovine growth hormone, so look for labels stating No rBGH, rBST, or artificial hormones. If you live in Europe, avoiding GM foods is easier because laws require labelling.

By avoiding GMOs, you become part of the tipping point of consumer rejection and the inevitable demise of this unnatural and dangerous element in our food supply. That tipping point may be closer than you think. It is already a liability to have to label food as such. The tipping point has been reached in Europe, where such food is despised and largely banned. We need to ensure it does not creep back in there. In countries where corporations still have a greater say than human beings, we need to keep the pressure up.

————

The GMO chapter could also be the Organic chapter. If you eat only organic foods, then by definition you will avoid GMOs. However, the case against GMOs is stronger than is the case for organic food. Let's face it, organic food can be expensive. It can be hard to find and hard to verify that it is indeed pesticide and GMO free. But in the end, it is up to you decide whether exiting GMO and 'eating like a hippie' is worth the effort and cost.

I now avoid GMOs like the plague. I wouldn't say I can physically detect the difference to my health or well-being. But when I see anything or read anything about GMOs and knowing what I know now, I'm thankful that I don't go near that crap. What I can notice physically, however, is the effect of minimal processed food in my belly. In my effort to quit GMOs I have stopped shopping in supermarkets. I favour organic supplies wherever possible. Food has become more treasured. I don't take healthy, natural food for granted, and I maybe even eat a little less in general. I know exactly what I have in my fridge or pantry, value the preparation and consumption of each meal a lot more, and I have zero waste food. I'm not going to let vegetables that have consumed so much effort and cash to find and buy go to waste.

In the same way that 'meat' commoditises animals and erodes our empathy for them, I've realised that supermarket shopping commoditises 'food'. We tend to care very little about what it is, where it came from, how much we need, and whether it is wasted or not. This is what is keeping us alive, folks. It needs to be a more thoughtful and important part of our lives. It's time to stop eating what you are dished up, push your plate away from the table, and say, "No more corn for me!" And then you can demand the food that your body will thank you for.

ACTIONS

•Watch *GMO OMG*, an amazing documentary exposing the truth about GMOs **http://www.gmofilm.com.**

•Watch *Bitter Seeds* to find out about the Indian GMO failure **http://teddybearfilms.fatcow.com/2011/10/01/bitter-seeds-2.**

•Locate nearby organic produce markets and suppliers.

•Replace supermarket processed 'crap' with organic 'food' on Liberation Day.

•De-risk your health in the process.

MENU

Do Eat	Eat in Moderation	Eat If You Must	Do Not Eat
Fresh, local whole foods Opt for certified organic or labelled GMO Free	Animal based products labelled grass-fed or organic so that you know they were not raised on GMO feed	Food from a supermarket Suspect ingredients such whey, xanthan gum, glutamate, hydrolysed vegetable protein, lactic acid, cellulose, citric acid, maltodextrin, and diglycerides	Known GMO crops and foods in your country

WEEK 10 - DAIRY

"The human body has no more need for cow's milk than it does for dog's milk, horse's milk or giraffe's milk."

—Michael Klaper, MD

———

Let's imagine a parallel universe in which our species evolved in a manner that saw us consuming milk and yogurt made from almonds, soybeans, and coconuts, eating butter-like substances made from natural oils, and eating cheese made from nuts. Now picture some clever humanoid claiming that all of these nutritious foods could be sourced from one animal. Ears would prick up, wouldn't they?

The ensuing conversation would expose a few minor drawbacks. To produce these foods, the animal in question would require ten times the resources compared to the existing plant-based sources. Vast amounts of biodiverse land would need to be cleared, which together with this animals' potent methane-loaded farts would result in the single biggest contributor to climate change. There would be a minor issue of having to torture said animal to make it profitable. As the products from this animal would not be as nutritious as the current products in use, and most likely hazardous, it would be necessary to fabricate some health benefits and market the hell out of them so people would consume them. Oh, and lastly, everyone would need to effectively breastfeed off of another mammal, even as adults. Still sound okay? Attention would quickly wane. Phone calls to mental asylums would be made.

I believe in making choices based on free will every day of my life. I look at how I want life to be, and then I do what I can to live in to that reality. I don't necessarily use what is the historical norm as a reference. It is a lot easier and more effective to focus on creating a new 'now' from scratch than the messy and cumbersome process of modifying the old.

So, each day my 'now' is faced with a similar decision to the one put forward in the parallel universe. Do I choose to eat these foods from the plant-based sources or choose the animal-based source with all of its massive drawbacks as outlined in the parallel universe? What do you think? All of history and all of the reality of our actual universe aside, wouldn't you strongly reject the animal-based source?

WHAT IS DAIRY?

When I initially climbed into this subject, I had the idea that the result would be some kind of hybrid cleanse, removing only the worst and leaving some of the good dairy on my plate. Once I'd finished the research, however, and once I had an understanding of all the aspects and the scale of dairy's negative impact on me and the planet, I decided to eliminate all dairy, even cheese. Ouch! I have provided a soft-core option in

The Cleanse section because I know how tough this is, but I'll carry on in hard-core 'no dairy' mode for now.

In a nutshell, a dairy product is food produced from the milk of mammals. This includes milk itself, milk-based yogurt, cheese, butter, and cream. As for ice cream, if I didn't persuade you to drop it in previous chapters, maybe I'll get you with this one.

HOW MUCH DO WE CONSUME AND WHY?

Milk is much more than just a drink. It is a cultural phenomenon that can be traced back thousands of years. The need and reasons for drinking it since then may have changed, but the animal milk myth is as strong as ever. According to the UN's Food and Agriculture Organization:

Based on milk equivalent (ME), average per capita global milk consumption amounts to about 100 kg of milk/year, with very significant differences between countries/regions. Per capita consumption in Western Europe is in excess of 300 kg of milk/ year compared with less than 30 kg (and even sometimes as little as 10 kg) in some African and Asian countries. It may be expected that increasing income levels will stimulate the demand for milk and dairy products.[71]

More than 6 billion people worldwide consume non-human milk and milk products, most of whom live in developing countries. Since the 1960s per capita milk consumption in developing countries has doubled. However, the consumption of milk has grown more slowly than the consumption of meat (tripled) and eggs (fivefold increase).

————————

Humans are the only earth species that consumes milk in adulthood and the only species that does so from the 'udder of another mammal's mudda'. The function of cow's milk is to feed a rapidly growing calf, to beef it up (pun unavoidable). If we are not calves and we do not need fattening up, then why the heck are we drinking cows' milk? Pretty weird, if you ask me. If we are going to drink milk as adults, shouldn't it at least be human milk? I put it down to three main reasons.

1. **Marketing.** We continue to consume milk without question largely due to the massive marketing effort that convinces us that it is beneficial and indeed necessary in our diet. Clearly, that we "need" baby cow food is utter nonsense regardless of whether there are health benefits. One of the world's best-ever marketing ploys tells us milk is wholesome and nutritious. Cow food has even managed to make its way into the human 'food pyramid'! We are constantly advised that milk is part of a healthy diet, provides essential nutrients, strengthens our bones, and prevents osteoporosis. Even if this were true, which it is not, it doesn't mean we need to drink it. Engulfing yourself for a short while in flames leaving third degree burns all over your body will indeed prevent unwanted hair growth, but this does not mean it is a satisfactory approach to hair removal.

2. **The calcium myth.** One of the alleged core truths used by the milk marketing machine is that humans need to consume calf food because the calcium in it will maintain strong bones and prevent osteoporosis. This fanciful nonsense has been drilled into us since childhood. The basis for milk's promotion is that it contains about 300mg per cup. But that doesn't mean the calcium ends up in our bones. The fact is that we barely absorb the calcium in cow's milk, especially if pasteurised. Worse still and mildly ironic, the ingestion of cow's milk actually increases calcium loss from bones. I'll explain how this happens in the next section, but this finding is supported by statistics that show that countries with the lowest consumption of dairy products also have the lowest fracture incidences in their population.

3. **Cheese is addictive.** By now you must be asking what isn't addictive? Well, I hate to be the bearer of more bad news, but the casein in dairy releases opiates called casomorphins, which are similar to morphine. This makes a lot of sense when you consider the purpose of mother's milk is to provide nourishment for rapidly growing infants and establish a strong connection between mother and child. It's biologically intelligent to have babies addicted to mothers' milk. Cheese, made primarily from cow's milk, concentrates the casomorphins by about ten times compared to milk, making it very addictive indeed! Don't fret, though, you won't need to go to rehab or follow a 12-step program to quit cheese, but it's good to be aware of why you crave it. It's not just because it tastes awesome.

Why Is Dairy Bad?

T. Colin Campbell and Thomas M. Campbell's *The China Study,* the largest comprehensive study of human nutrition ever conducted, surmises that dairy consumption is far worse for us than we think.[72] It can lead to numerous health issues.

1. **Excessive marketing**. Don't you think that if something requires continual, excessive marketing, the product is not good enough to sell itself? Could there be issues with the product that continuously need masking?

2. **The calcium myth continued.** When you consume dairy, it, along with soda, processed fats, and animal protein, actually acidify the body's ph. This triggers the body to neutralise the acid by using calcium from the body's most abundant source, the bones. So the very calcium that we are told is needed to keep our bones strong is used to neutralise the acidic effect of milk. Then the calcium leaves the body through the urine with the end result being a net deficit in bodily calcium. You don't see that in milk advertisements, now, do you?

   There is plenty of research to support this claim, such as the comprehensive, twelve-year "Harvard Nurses' Health Study",[73] which started in 1989 and followed more than 75,000 women. Not only did it show absolutely no protective effect of dairy on bones, it also revealed an increased risk of hip fracture in old age.[74]

   Even human breast milk is not that great a source of calcium. Nuts and certain vegetables contain high calcium content and do not have an overall acidic effect in the body like milk does. As such they are more conducive to calcium retention.

3. **Inflammation**. Dairy causes inflammation in a large per cent of the population, resulting in digestive issues such as bloating, gas, constipation, and diarrhoea.

4. **Lactose intolerance.** The main carbohydrate in dairy is lactose, a sugar made up of glucose and galactose. Babies produce an enzyme called lactase that breaks down this lactose. But many people lose the ability to do that in adulthood.[75] This applies to about three quarters of the world's population.[76]

5. **Hormones and antibiotics**. The United States and Brazil are the only countries that inject cows with the genetically engineered bovine growth hormone rBGH to increase milk yield. It's so vile that it is banned in most countries. The forced increase in milk production regularly leads to udder infections known as mastitis, which are treated with antibiotics, which then can make their way into your dairy products. Antibiotics are also used for other cow ailments.

6. **Fattening.** What is milk designed for? It's designed to fatten up babies. Cow's milk is designed to fatten a calf into a 1,000-kilogram cow. If you want to lose weight, you wouldn't drink something that is designed to fatten something up as fast as possible, would you?

7. **Eczema and acne.** Quitting dairy is the best thing you can do for your skin. Hormones in cows' milk cause eczema, acne, redness, and soreness in the skin. Milk also causes excess oil production in the skin, which is not good for any of these conditions.[77]

8. **Cancer.** These same hormones have been linked to colon, pancreas, endometrium, breast, and prostate cancer.[78] Ovarian cancer has also been linked.[79]

9. **Animal cruelty.** The impact on humans can be massive, but it pales in comparison to the wretched lives that dairy cows lead. The cows that are raised for dairy are generally forced to live in atrocious conditions. They are continuously and mechanically made pregnant for their entire lives from around twelve months of age. Their babies are taken away from them at birth, which is traumatising for both the mother and the calf. A normal cow lives for twenty or more years, but dairy cows are usually turned into meat after they collapse from the exhaustion of permanent pregnancy at around five years old. If they don't collapse, their production goes down at that age so they are turned into burgers anyway. So it's like the miserable life of a beef cow, preceded by sexual and emotional torture for five years. Think about that. In her YouTube clip, Erin Janus convincingly tells us about how we inflict all of this misery on a fellow earthling so that we can consume something that we simply do not need to consume.[80]

10. **Environment**. And finally, a dairy cow is still a cow, and so all of the environmental issues that I discussed in the Land-Based Meat chapter apply to dairy cows as well.

THE CLEANSE

The decision to quit dairy came down to my conscience and to my body. I've found that from a health perspective it's absolutely not needed in the human diet, and I believe it has a negative influence on the body when you weigh the pros and cons. That being the case, the only reason I would eat dairy is for taste. Cheese is yummy. Add to that rationale the whole animal cruelty factor, and the question then becomes whether or not I am happy to be responsible for animal torture to satisfy my taste buds. The answer to that is a resounding no. Armed with my alternatives to dairy below, I won't be eating any dairy.

Here is where the soft-core option comes into play. Given that ultimately the question comes down to taste versus torture, if you can source dairy that is made from raw milk from an organic grass-fed animal, ideally from a local small holding, then you have some wiggle room. Such dairy contains loads more nutrients and live enzymes than pasteurised products. And then full-fat mitigates some of the insulin spike and makes the calcium more easily accessible. Typically, this comes from farms that treat animals more humanely because profit is not their sole motive.

So, start by eliminating all dairy and notice how you feel. Then as needed, source organic grass-fed dairy only and allow that in your diet if you must. If you take the hard-core option, do not fear; there are plenty of alternatives and many sources of calcium that run rings around dairy.

If still you're umming and ahhing about the need to address dairy, take a look at *Farmageddon* for a realistic eye opener about what your appetite for dairy does to other sentient beings of this earth. [81]

————

I've left the door open to eat dairy under certain conditions. Who knows? I may even nibble on a bit of cheese or munch down some Greek yogurt myself if I can verify its source. In line with that, I'll include in these replacements the best options in the soft-core quitting category.

1. **Raw milk.** If you are determined to drink cow's milk then drink organic, full-fat, raw milk from cows fed on grass. These cows have not been injected with rGBH and have not been treated with antibiotics. Raw milk still contains many of the helpful enzymes that the pasteurisation process destroys. This includes the lactase enzyme that breaks down lactose, meaning folks who are lactose intolerant can drink it without issue. What applies to raw cow's milk applies also to raw goat and sheep's milk and to all dairy products that are made from it.

2. **Milk from nuts.** The best alternatives to milk from mammals is milk from nuts. Almonds, cashews, hazelnuts, Brazil nuts, and coconut milk are all great sources of calcium and are generally alkalising so they do not leach calcium from your body. Hazelnuts have loads of vitamin E and are good for hair and skin. Coconut milk is free of dairy, soy, lactose, gluten, casein, and MSG, but it also has no protein.

3. **Other milk.** You also have milk from hemp, oats, rice and soy. Make sure your soy beans are not GMO.

4. **Raw milk yogurt.** The best dairy-based yogurt option is made from organic, full-cream, raw milk. Stay away from low fat and flavoured versions. They are borderline junk food and contain lots of sugar. Depending on what's available near you, go for natural or Greek varieties.

5. **Coconut yogurt.** There is really no need to chase raw milk yogurt as you can avoid dairy altogether and buy or make coconut yogurt. I'm talking about yogurt made from coconuts, not coconut-flavoured yogurt. It's full of the good fats of the coconut so you will feel fuller sooner. You can add lemon to make it taste a bit more like Greek yogurt and add fresh fruit as you like.

6. **Cheese.** This is the hardest one to replace primarily because cheese tastes so damn good. Unfortunately, I do not have a replacement that is quite as tasty, but that's one of the only costs of avoiding dairy. I suspect I'll crack and need to eat some cheese at some point, but I'll make sure it's from raw, organic milk. You can get some vegan cheeses made from nuts and seeds. Check out speciality and health food stores. I recently made a cheese cake using a cashew 'cheese' foundation, and it was actually quite good. The Internet has loads of such recipes.

7. **Ice cream.** I did not expect to still be eating ice cream once I quit dairy. A quick search of the Internet revealed loads of companies that make a dairy-free version of ice cream. I have started making my own just to prove the point and am having a lot of success using coconut milk, dates, almond milk, and cacao or fresh fruit. I used a few recipes collected by the Academy of Culinary Nutrition to get me started.[82]

8. **Other calcium sources.** Just in case you're still not convinced that you will get enough calcium if you ditch dairy, there's plenty of plant-based food that will fill that gap. For fruit and vegetables eat oranges, figs, olives, spinach, kale and other dark leafy greens, collard greens, broccoli, and red kidney beans. Sesame seeds, quinoa,

chia seeds, Brazil nuts, and tofu are also good sources, as are sardines and salmon with bones in a can.

————

With land-based meat already stricken from my diet, removing dairy means I no longer have a need for cows. Cows really are the scourge when it comes to the environment whether it is from land clearing or their methane farts. I do rant sometimes about these two environmental concerns, so by not personally adding to the human demand for cows, I feel like I'm standing on more solid ground when I say that cows suck.

Living in Indonesia it is quite easy to avoid dairy, as there's not a lot of it around anyway. But knowing what is in my milk and how it's produced, I think I'd struggle to consume it anyway if I were in the West. It is so bad for you and our earth. I know acquired habits die as hard as acquired tastes, but the move away from this type of food production has no choice but to happen. Without trying to sound dramatic, the alternate choice is eventual global death for one and all. This move is achievable. The move towards the current dairy situation happened, so the move away can happen too.

If each dairy-munching earthling migrates to the alternatives provided, demand will slowly die, just like demand slowly grew. When demand dies at an exponential rate as the truth becomes more widespread, cows that die won't be replaced. This is the terminal butt cork for the global cow herd. Methane from cow farts will wane. The forest that was laid to waste to host cows can grow back, and we can look forward to a living planet, not a dying one.

ACTIONS

•Watch You Tube clip:
https://www.youtube.com/watch?v=UcN7SGGoCNI.

•Watch *Farmageddon*
https://www.youtube.com/watch?v=2rLeozMRLOs.

•Locate nearby organic, raw milk from grass-fed animals in case you need it.

•Stop eating all dairy initially to check out how you feel.

•Use replacements and only introduce actual dairy if you can verify the source.

MENU

Do Eat	Eat in Moderation	Eat If You Must	Do Not Eat
Milk from almonds, cashews, hazelnuts, brazil nuts, coconuts, hemp, oats, rice, and GMO-free soy

Coconut yoghurt

Vegan cheese made from nuts and seeds

Dairy-free ice cream | | Organic, full-fat, raw milk from cows, goats, and sheep fed on grass and derivatives of this

Greek yoghurt from organic raw milk | Milk, milk-based yogurt, cheese, butter. and cream made from milk of mammals |

WEEK 11 - SEAFOOD

"I don't eat fish because there is no such thing as sustainable fishing right now."

—Paul Watson

————————

Sharks kill twelve people per year; people kill 11,417 sharks per hour. Folks, in this consumption cleanse we may well be running out of stuff to eat here, but why are we finning sharks just because certain people have small ... feet? I accept I might lose a lot of readers from that comment, but as at the time of writing I only have twenty-nine Facebook followers, so I am going to run with it. Killing a top predator on the false hope that we might wear bigger socks one day is bad enough, but to dump the then-mutilated body almost in its entirety back into the sea is a disgraceful waste to boot.

WHAT IS SEAFOOD?

I believe and accept that seafood used to be a part of a healthy and balanced diet. Whether it is healthy to catch and eat seafood nowadays is debatable. My approach to this category is more convoluted than are other chapters because I'll be picking and choosing certain seafood items to eat based on their impact on human and planetary health.

Fish from depleted and over-fished fisheries or from those that use fishing methods with a large bycatch are excluded from my diet. Anything that is likely to have high mercury or PCB (polychlorinated biphenyls, industrial products, or chemicals) content is also off the menu. And I won't be eating any seafood from large chain supermarkets or that is imported, in particular from anywhere close to the Fukushima nuclear disaster zone or its subsequent growing radiation plume.

Specifically, what species does this cleanse exclude?

Large-scale fisheries are often vulnerable because they target the larger marine animals that have a longer life and are slow to reproduce. These animals are also found higher in the food chain and as such have been ingesting more mercury and PCBs for longer, so they are not good for you anyway. This category includes bluefin, yellow fin, and albacore tuna, orange roughy, halibut, shark, swordfish, marlin, Spanish and king mackerel, sea bass, grouper, and tilefish. These are the big ones to avoid. For a comprehensive list of seafood and its mercury content, I have included a table in "Why Is Seafood Bad?" What mostly remains on my plate are small, fast-to-reproduce species that are neither endangered nor loaded with mercury, such as anchovies and sardines.

Of the fish that have a poor bycatch record, mahi mahi, and shrimp take the cake. Shrimp is a tough one because it tastes so good, but in most cases wild-caught shrimp comes from bottom-trawling, which takes a heavy toll on other sea life.

Farmed fish includes ocean and land-based farms. If you cannot verify that it is wild-caught, assume it is farmed. Salmon, excluding Alaskan wild-caught, is usually farmed as are panga, tilapia, carp, bass, sturgeon, trout, and shrimp.

In terms of other shell fish, I'll take guidance from the Safina Center's seafood guide.[83]

And watch out for seaweed and kelp from around Japan and China. It's probably radioactive.

HOW MUCH DO WE CONSUME AND WHY?

The amount of seafood we earthlings consume over and above what is sustainable is huge.

According to Michael D'Orso and Ted Danson, "In 55 years human have managed to wipe out 90% of the oceans top predators. These are animals like sharks, Bluefin tuna, swordfish, marlin, and king mackerel."[84]

According to the National Geographic Society, "By 1989, when about 90 million metric tons of catch were taken from the ocean, the industry had hit its high-water mark, and yields have declined or stagnated ever since."[85]

According to Oceana.org, "Aquaculture, or fish farming, requires feed for captive fish. To grow just one pound of farmed salmon, an estimated four to eleven pounds of prey fish are consumed. As the aquaculture industry continues to expand, prey fish are depleted at alarming and unsustainable rates. If current trends continue, some researchers predict that aquaculture will outgrow the supply of fishmeal as soon as 2020."[86]

And according to the UN FAO, "Americans now eat four times as much seafood as we did 50 years ago, but fish populations have not been able to keep up with our increasing appetites. By conservative estimates, about 32% of world fish stocks are estimated to be overexploited, depleted, or desperately in need of respite and recovery, according to the Food and Agriculture Organization."[87]

—————

We all know that fish are an important part of a balanced diet, a top source of protein and omega-3s, and taste great. This is why we eat fish. We've always eaten fish. But we haven't always had the dire situation that we now have in the oceans. We need to look again and see if there are any reasons to eat fish today.

Other than for a very few exceptions, I would say that there are not.

WHY IS SEAFOOD BAD?

The massive increase in global seafood consumption and the advent of "factory fish farming" have fundamentally changed the oceanic environment and the very nature of fish as a food. Seafood has gone from being abundant and healthy to being on the verge of ecological collapse and toxic. If you are not eating seafood intelligently, then you are most likely an accomplice to the poisoning of the earth and your own body. Following is a list of the big issues with seafood.

1. **By catch.** Destructive fishing practises greatly contribute to avoidable depopulation of sea life. Large-scale fishing produces loads of accidental bycatch that is simply dumped at sea, dead or dying. Bottom trawling, the worst offender accounting for 50% of global bycatch, drags nets across the ocean floor to catch shrimp. This kills large numbers of marine life not targeted like crabs and young fish: 26 pounds of bycatch perish for each one pound of shrimp caught. Long-lining and gill netting are also destructive methods, particularly for sea turtles, with over 28,000 caught in shrimp nets every year. Additionally, 300,000 whales, dolphins, and porpoises die each year from getting snagged as bycatch.[88]

2. **Mercury.** Activities such as coal burning and iron mining contaminate water sources with methyl mercury. This is then absorbed into the bodies of fish. This dangerous neurotoxin affects brain function and the nervous system and is extremely dangerous to young children and pregnant women. Generally, the higher up in the oceanic food chain and the longer the lifespan of the animal, the greater the concentration of mercury. This is simply because big fish eat little fish, and older fish do so for longer. So short-lived seafood low in the food chain, such as squid, scallops, and

sardines, has less mercury than top predators like tuna and swordfish. The table below from *The Smart Seafood Buying Guide* shows us which sea life is the most dangerous in terms of mercury.[89]

LEAST MERCURY	MODERATE MERCURY	HIGH MERCURY	HIGHEST MERCURY
Enjoy these fish	Eat six servings or less per month	Eat three servings or less per month	Avoid eating
Anchovies	Bass (Saltwater, Striped, Black)	Croaker (White Pacific)	Bluefish
Butterfish	Buffalofish	Halibut (Atlantic, Pacific)	Grouper
Catfish	Carp	Mackerel (Spanish, Gulf)	Mackerel (King)
Clam	Cod (Alaskan)	Perch (Ocean)	Marlin
Crab (Domestic)	Lobster	Sablefish	Orange Roughy
Crawfish/Crayfish	Mahi Mahi	Sea Bass (Chilean)	Shark
Croaker (Atlantic)	Monkfish	Tuna (Albacore, Yellowfin)	Swordfish
Flounder	Perch (Freshwater)		Tuna (Bigeye, Ahi)
Haddock (Atlantic)	Sheepshead		
Hake	Skate		
Herring	Snapper		
Jacksmelt (Silverside)	Tilefish (Atlantic)		
Mackerel	Tuna (Canned chunk light, Skipjack)		
(N. Atlantic, Chub)			
Mullet			
Oyster			
Plaice			
Pollock			
Salmon (Canned)			
Salmon (Fresh)			
Sardine			
Scallop			
Shrimp			
Sole (Pacific)			
Squid (Calamari)			
Tilapia			
Trout (Freshwater)			
Whitefish			
Whiting			

3. **PCBs and other toxins.** Most major waterways are loaded with heavy metals, dioxins, PCBs, and other agricultural chemicals that wind up in the environment. These make their way into the seafood we eat, and it doesn't take a nuclear scientist to know that they are not good things to be putting in the water or your body.

4. **Fukushima radiation.** Speaking of nuclear scientists, why are they not speaking out about this one? A

Canadian high school student named Bronwyn Delacruz was surprised to discover radioactive fish in a school science project with a gifted $600 Geiger counter. She ran her radiation detector over seafood bought at her local store and discovered that a lot of the Chinese products sent her machine spinning. It made the headlines and got people talking. It turns out that most governments, while they used to test for radiation in the wake of the 2011 Fukushima nuclear disaster, decided to stop testing around 2012. How odd.

"Some of the kelp that I found was higher than what the International Atomic Energy Agency sets as radioactive contamination, which is 1,450 counts over a 10-minute period," Bronwyn said. "Some of my samples came up as 1,700 or 1,800."

Back in 2012, the *Vancouver Sun* reported that cesium-137 was being found in a very high per cent of the fish that Japan was selling to Canada.[90] Another test off the Californian coast found all 15 out of 15 Bluefin tuna tested were contaminated with Fukushima radiation.[91] And I found plenty more independent and verified tests showing high levels of radioactivity in Pacific Ocean fish.

5. **Farmed fish.** When you can't manage a better solution, there is farmed fish, which can be done either with open net pens in the water or land-based pens. Both are no good for you, but the latter is not as bad for the planet. The majority of fish farms are bounded by open-net pens in the ocean where tightly packed fish stagnate over a mountain of their own waste teeming with bacteria, drugs, and pesticides, which drifts unchecked into the open ocean. The overcrowding almost always

results in infection with parasites and disease, frequently spreading to and decimating wild fish populations, which have to be treated with ever-increasing doses of antibiotics. In addition, the farmed fish are pumped full of chemicals to make them grow faster and have a more consumable colour. All of this junk makes its way to the sea floor and devastates everything there.

Aquaculture tells us that it's the solution to the fishery depletion problem, but in fact it is blatantly and knowingly making it much worse. It takes between three and eleven pounds of wild fish to grow one pound of salmon. Fish farms are the leading cause of mangrove destruction. They marginalise local communities and leech invasive species and pollutants into the surrounding areas. And as for the fish coming out of these farms, well, they are some of the most toxic things you can put in your body. Farmed fish have ten times the cancer-causing organic pollutants that wild fish have, are much higher in saturated fats, and have lower levels of beneficial omega-3 fatty acids than wild fish. The fish feed contains chicken shit. What the hell? This stuff is not a health food.

A great documentary by Nicolas Daniel called *"Fillet Oh Fish"* smashes the romantic myth of fish farming and exposes this industry for what it is.[92]

6. **Imported seafood.** Besides the obvious environmental and economic cost of transportation, the lack of control around sustainable fisheries in export countries tells me to steer clear. Chemical use, environmental destruction, and human exploitation are usually far worse than what is acceptable in Western countries. I

found out that imported shrimp from Thailand is filthy, often found to contain huge levels of antibiotics, rat and mouse hair, unauthorised chemical residues, and even pieces of insects.

7. **Big-box stores.** These are the massive supermarket chains. They are listed companies. Profit is god. Sea life welfare and environmental and health considerations are meaningless. Do not buy seafood from these places. They will be the first to accept GMO 'monster fish' based on cost and their affiliation with biotech companies. Call me a fear monger but do your own research. The web of inter-company affiliation is surprisingly opaque, and 90% of frozen fish in big-box stores comes from fish farms.

THE CLEANSE

Eating seafood that is both healthful and sustainable comes down to moderation and education. Moderation is subjective, but once you have educated yourself, there won't be that much seafood to eat anyway unless you can eat anchovies and sardines all day every day.

Education is ongoing regarding the oceans, and fisheries are constantly changing, so you need to set yourself up with a few basic tools to stay on top of things. First is the knowledge that the most sustainable and healthful seafood is eaten in moderation, responsibly harvested, local, and low on the food chain. Second, I keep my eye on publications like the seafood guide from The Safina Center. I also have a smartphone app to which I refer if I'm unsure about certain seafood. Monterey Bay

Aquarium's Seafood Watch app is free, so there's no excuse, and it's smart enough to use your current location to tell you what is safe where you are.

————————

There is plenty of information above to know what is not good to eat. Here's a list of seafood that at the time of writing still finds its way into my belly.

1. **Tiny fishes.** Smaller species that reproduce early in life, have short life spans, and are an abundant, strong, and fertile part of the food chain include anchovies, herring, and sardines. These diminutive fish are super tasty and high in good oils and omega-3s. Anchovies are rich in iron. Sardines are naturally high in vitamin D.

2. **Wild-caught Alaskan salmon.** Both steak and canned versions are packed with omega-3s. The canned version is a great source of calcium due to the bony bits in it. It comes from an extremely well-managed fishery to the point of having biologists stationed at the river mouths counting the fish that return for spawning. If numbers dwindle, they slash quotas. It's also low in contaminants like lead and mercury. Alaskan salmon is not allowed to be farmed.

3. **Bivalve shellfish.** Mussels, oysters, and clams are often good options as they are the most likely seafood items at restaurants or markets to be sustainably sourced. They are filter feeders, so they help to improve local environments by cleaning up water, even in farms. But

this does mean they may also be taking in lots of contaminants, so ask about local contaminant warnings first.

For me, that's it. That's the only seafood I eat.

––––––

This all might sound a bit constrictive, but there's a positive side that I prefer to focus on with seafood. By no longer eating most seafood and being very selective when I do, I am certainly doing my body a huge favour. Sure, I take a bit more time to find something to eat, but when I do come across wild-caught Alaskan salmon I get a bit excited, and I enjoy the hell out of it. Fresh sardines have always been a favourite of mine, and I'm finding more and more ways to turn the contents of the humble sardine can into something delicious.

Other than having no more seaborne toxic chemicals going into my body, the biggest personal benefit for me is pizza. With what was left for me to eat at this stage of the cleanse, the pizza situation was starting to look a bit grim. Pizza for me was a baseless, meatless, cheeseless arrangement of a few organic vegetables scattered around a plate of unconfined tomato sauce. Your average punter would not see pizza there, but if you add anchovies . . .

And as for all the other seafood I no longer eat for environmental reasons, a lot of the bigger varieties have toxic levels of mercury inside of them anyway. Whether I saw myself as an entity apart from the natural world or as a part of it, I see reasons to act out of self-interest and cease consuming it.

ACTIONS

•Watch the *Fillet Oh Fish* documentary to inspire this dietary shift **https://www.youtube.com/watch?v=MgrFXN4d1Jc.**

•Print the guide from The Blue Ocean Institute so you know what not to eat
http://www.safinacenter.org/files/Seafood_Guide.pdf

•Get the Seafood Watch app on your smartphone.

•Restrict your seafood consumption on Liberation Day.

•Give the fisheries and your body a chance to recover.

MENU

Do Eat	Eat in Moderation	Eat If You Must	Do Not Eat
Small, short-lived fish such as anchovies, herring, and sardines Bivalve shellfish	Wild-caught Alaskan salmon	Local medium-sized fish caught sustainably from fisheries not listed as at risk	All farmed fish All large fish with slow reproductive cycles and longer lives such as tuna, shark, swordfish, mackerel, and tilefish. Fish caught in China, Japan and other areas affected by the Fukushima disaster

WEEK 12 - FOOD ADDITIVES

"The food you eat can be either the safest and most powerful form of medicine or the slowest form of poison."

—Ann Wigmore

————

It is today's children who will suffer most at the hands of the vast expansion of additives in processed food. If you have children, you need to read this. If you are short on time, go straight to the Cleanse and just use the other sections as a reference, but do not ignore this chapter.

Oh, for the days of yore when farmers grew food and then we ate it. Now food is grown by businessmen in chemical fields designed for profit, not nutrition. The scientists have also gotten hold of it and 'cooked' it in a lab so that this pseudo-food is even further away from what nature intended and what our bodies need. Food manufacturers then chemically modify the pseudo-food into a 'hardly-food' by adding a chemical cocktail of additives. This process adds to the shelf life and the appearance of the food. But it subtracts from the shelf life and appearance of the consumer, particularly children.

If you've got children, then this chapter is for you. Grab a cup of green tea, buckle up, and get ready for a chemistry lesson.

WHAT ARE FOOD ADDITIVES?

Here I'll cover chemically produced artificial colours, flavour enhancers, preservatives, and a few other additives that I try to avoid. Most of them I no longer encounter because of all of the stuff I've already quit. I'll cover the worst of them, in case you've strayed from The Cleanse. Artificial sweeteners are food additives, but I've given them the hard time they deserve in earlier chapters.

1. **Artificial colours**. Made from chemicals in a lab, artificial colours and dyes have no nutritional value. They are for cosmetic purposes used to increase sales. Most of them have detrimental health effects which I discuss below. They are found in foods like cordials, condiments, lollies, cakes, sausages, and soft drinks.

2. **Flavour enhancers**. These cheap chemical mixtures that mimic natural flavours include glutamates (including monosodium glutamate or MSG) and are found in loads of food such as packet soups, flavoured noodles, sauces, and savoury snacks. When this stuff hits the tongue, it gives food a savoury taste. But as MSG has such a bad name, food manufacturers either use other sources of glutamates such as protein extracts from corn or the yeast

of soy. Alternatively, they simply call it something else such as autolysed vegetable protein, autolysed yeast, hydrolysed vegetable protein, and yeast extract. It is frequently found in other ingredients like maltodextrin, sodium caseinate, and even citric acid where it is not required to be listed as a separate ingredient. Sounds yummy, doesn't it?

3. **Preservatives.** This category includes nitrites and nitrates used to extend the shelf life of meat by keeping it from going rancid and slowing bacteria growth. Typically these are found in processed and cured meats like ham, hot dogs, sausage, and bacon. Sulphites including sulphur dioxide act as preservatives to prevent bacterial growth. They are found in beer, soft drinks, dried fruits, juices, cordials, wine, vinegar, and potato products. Sorbates preserve food without changing its taste, smell, or colour and prevent yeast from growing. Benzoates such as tert-Butylhydroquinone (TBHQ) butylatedhydroxyanisole (BHA), and butylatedhydroxytoluene (BHT) are preservatives made from coal tar and butane and are found in cereals, chewing gum, potato chips, and vegetable oils. They keep foods from changing colour, changing flavour, and becoming rancid. Other benzoates include benzoic acid, sodium benzoates, potassium benzoates, and calcium. Benzoates are used in fruit juices, carbonated drinks, and pickles to stymie the growth of microorganisms in acidic foods. Are you feeling like you might need a chemistry degree just to eat healthy foods?

4. **Other additives.** Diacetyl is added to butter in microwave popcorn. Aluminium is an additive in baking powder and anti-caking agents. Potassium bromate is

used to increase the volume of white flour, breads, and rolls such as in the not-so-wonderful Wonder Bread.

HOW MUCH DO WE CONSUME AND WHY?

Across the Western world between 70–90% of the household food budget is allocated to processed food, which is food that's not really just food anymore. Almost all processed food uses some kind of additives, whether it's a colouring, a preservative, or who knows what?

Based on the US Food and Drug Administration database, there are some 3,000 different things "added to food in the United States."[93] A thousand such items in the database contain no other information or qualitative data than simple administrative details. I'm not suggesting that every country has the same quantity of known additives, but this is a massive number! Is food as it is grown and meant to be, by nature, that bad that we need this many additives?

————

No, the reason we consume so many additives in our food is simple. We eat mostly processed food instead of real food for convenience, and most processed food contains additives to boost sales and shelf life, lower costs or all of the above. Food itself does not need additives. The lubricant that helped this current situation to slide out of control is the lack of consumer education about the dangers of additives. Without consumer resistance, the profit motive fuels the need to keep things on the shelf for longer, make them easier to market, and entice you to eat more of them. As consumers we need to wise up.

WHY ARE FOOD ADDITIVES BAD?

Food additives are an unnecessary chemical evil. If you can avoid all processed food and eat only organic, vegetarian, whole foods, you'll be almost safe from them, but you'll still need to stay alert. This stuff creeps into everything.

1. **Artificial colours.** An increase in ADHD diagnoses is widely blamed on the artificial colours in food. "It can affect their focus, their concentration. They become more easily distracted and become more impulsive. I think we're looking at a whole population of kids with skewed immune systems," says Dr Kenneth Bock,[94] who has studied at length the relationship between artificial colours and hyperactivity in children. The results of another study by the Centre for Science in the Public Interest finds connections between food colours Red 2(E123), Red 3(E127), Red 40(E129), Yellow 5(E102), and Yellow 6(E110) to cancer, chromosomal damage, lymphocytic lymphomas, and thyroid, lymph and kidney tumours.[95] The same study again finds that mixtures of dyes cause hyperactivity and other behavioural impairments in children. Other colours that have been identified as likely to be related to increased hyperactivity in children are tartrazine (E102), quinoline yellow (E104), sunset yellow FCF (E110), carmoisine (E122), ponceau 4R (E124), allura red AC (E129), amaranth

purple (E123), erythrosine cherry red (E127), indigo blue (E132), brilliant blue (E133), green (E142, E143), black (E151), and brown (E155). E107, E150, and E160(b) should also be avoided according to a comprehensive additives schedule produced by the Hyperactive Children's Support Group (HACSG).[96]

2. **Flavour enhancers.** Glutamates (E620–E625) are used by the food industry to keep you addicted to foods that, without them, you wouldn't eat in such quantities. They're substances that cause a Pavlovian trigger response to eat more. They've been shown to produce jaw aches, high blood pressure, nausea, fatigue, stomach ache, tight-jaw, dizziness, and chest pain.[97] MSG (E621), the bad boy poster child of the glutamates, can cause headaches, flushing, and numbness and exaggerate asthmatic symptoms. It is considered a neurotoxin because it overexcites nerve cells to the point of cell death.

3. **Nitrites.** Sodium nitrates and nitrites (E250 and E251) and potassium nitrites (E249 and E252) can lead to irritability, lack of energy, headaches, dizziness, pregnancy complications, and various infant health problems. All of these are listed as "probably carcinogenic to humans" by WHO's International Agency for Research on Cancer.[98]

4. **Sulphites.** Sulphites (E220, E221, E222 E223, E224, E225, E226, E227, and E228) can cause hay fever, runny nose, itchy eyes, and wheezing cough. About 10% of people will react with rashes, itching, restricted breathing, asthmatic attacks, hives or cramps. Sulphur dioxide (E220) can cause bronchial problems, low blood pressure, flushing and tingling sensations, and anaphylactic shock. It also kills vitamins B1 and E in the

body and is not recommended for consumption by children.[99] In fact, it's not recommended for consumption by anyone according to me.

5. **Sorbates.** Potassium sorbate (E202) and calcium sorbate (E203) are known to induce hypersensitivity in the mouth, throat, and eyes as well as migraines and headaches. Sorbic acid (E200) is probably a skin irritant.

6. **Benzoates.** TBHQ (319), BHA (320), and BHT (E321) are known carcinogens and yet are still not banned by some health authorities. They negatively affect the neurological system of the brain, sleep, and appetite. Consumption may also result in liver and kidney damage, hair loss, cancer, foetal abnormalities, and growth retardation. Is that enough for you? No? OK, they may also result in dizziness, hyperactivity, angioedema, asthma, rhinitis, dermatitis, and tumours and can affect oestrogen balance and levels. TBHQ may also cause nausea, vomiting, and delirium. A dose of 5g is considered fatal. How about now?

7. **More benzoates**. Benzoic acid (E210), sodium benzoate (E211), potassium benzoate (E212), and calcium benzoate (E213) are actually naturally occurring and mostly only affect people with allergies. However, when sodium benzoate is used in beverages also containing ascorbic acid (vitamin C), this results in small amounts of benzene. Benzene is a chemical that causes leukaemia.

8. **Diacetyl.** This popcorn additive is known to cause a serious condition called 'microwave popcorn lung'. Yes, I know this condition has a very cool name, but it can also cross the blood-brain barrier, a defence that prevents harmful substances from entering the brain. This can result in significant indications of Alzheimer's.

9. **Aluminium.** Aluminium is also widely suspected of contributing to Alzheimer's. Autopsies in the 1970s found many Alzheimer's sufferers contained high concentrations of aluminium in the brain.

10. **Potassium bromate**. This is known to cause cancer in animals. Luckily it is banned in every country except the United States and Japan because even small amounts of bread containing this substance can cause health problems.

THE CLEANSE

Additives and processed food go together. The more highly processed are the foods you eat; the more additives you'll eat. So, unless you have followed this cleanse verbatim, you can't easily avoid eating additives. The best thing you, and, more important, your children can do is to eat mainly fresh whole food. Alternatively, return to Chapter 1 and start again.

Start to make the shift in that direction. Start with the processed food that you feed your children. They tend to eat the same things regularly, so you need to check exactly what it is you are pumping into their little bodies each day. Can you eliminate it? Can you replace it with real food? If you cannot, then read the fine print on the packaging and see what additives are inside. Then cross-reference those additives with the list of ailments associated with those additives in "Why Are Food Additives Bad?" See if you are still happy for your kids to consume it. You can even try looking for competing processed products that do not contain so many additives.

Replicate the process for yourself by cross-examining the processed food you eat.

————————

Researching this topic for me was about supporting my decision to move away from processed foods and about knowing I'd dodged a bullet. It also gave me more fuel for the fire of my ranting when I spoke to people with children. I'm not completely supermarket free, but I have worked out for the items that I do still buy, which of these is the least bad of the options. Anything I buy that I am not familiar with gets the third-degree treatment so I know what additives are inside.

With this chapter there was no physical impact on me, and I wasn't expecting there to be one. I don't have any children, so they were also unaffected. I thought this chapter was necessary in order to be critical with processed foods if and when I do buy them. I hope it will also be useful to those who have picked and chosen some chapters of The Cleanse but not all of them and especially for folks with kids.

ACTIONS

•Look for opportunities to replace packaged food with real food.

•Analyse each item of processed food and compare additives to Why Are Food Additives Bad?

•Focus on your children's diet first and then yourself.

•Get a copy of the comprehensive Additives Schedule at **http://nac.allergyforum.com/additives/colors100-181.htm** and put it on your refrigerator.

MENU

Do Eat	Eat in Moderation	Eat If You Must	Do Not Eat
Fresh, organic, whole foods		Processed food that does not contain additives listed	Processed foods that contain artificial colours, particularly E123, E127, E129, E102, E107, E110, E104, E110, E122, E124, E129, E132, E133, E142, E143, E150, E151, E155, and 160b Processed foods that contain artificial flavours E620-E625 Processed foods that contain preservatives E250, E251, E249, E252, E220 – E228, E200, E202, E203, E319 - E321, and E210–E213

WEEK 13 - LESS IS MORE

"Eat less than you think you want, eat with your intelligence, not your stomach. Never get up from the table with an inward, silent apology for being a pig"

—Coco Chanel

———————

If I said there was a way for you to save money, lose weight, live healthier, and live longer and that to achieve it you just had to do less of something, would that whet your appetite?

We've all been bombarded by not only the content reflected in this book but also from every angle and through every type of mass media about what we should be eating. But what I am about to discuss is not about the components of your diet; it's not about telling you what to eat. This is about a far more fundamental and advantageous change you can make to your relationship to food. This is about eating less.

WHY EAT LESS?

I will confess to indulging in a feeding frenzy from time to time where I consume ridiculous amounts of food and drink. But eating better is the lifestyle ideal that I am continuously moving towards, not eating more. I'm convinced that while I may not live forever—in fact, I have serious doubts that I will—I will live longer and healthier by eating less. Eating too much is at the root of so many human and earthly problems that we have today. Simply eating less is one big step we can take to improve the health of body and globe.

Eating better has been covered in the previous chapters. This chapter is all about eating less.

1. **Reduced use of resources.** Eating less takes pressure off both global resources and your own. If you eat less the earth will need to produce less, you will need to buy less food, and you will need less money. If you need less money, you will need to work less, or at least you will have financial resources available for things that last longer.

2. **Longer life**. A growing body of research is showing why eating less and fasting add up to your living longer. In rodents, research has shown that low-calorie diets extended their lives by 30 to 40% compared to rodents eating standard diets.[100]

   Further up the food chain, a long-term study by the University of Wisconsin on Rhesus monkeys showed the calorie-restricted monkeys had far lower incidence of diabetes, heart and brain disease, and cancer than those eating more.[101] Dr Mosley from the BBC show *Horizon* tells us that it's the higher metabolic rates that lead us to earlier mortality. The metabolic rate measures how much energy the body uses for normal bodily functions such as eating: "The bottom line is that it is the only thing that's ever really been shown to prolong life. Ultimately, ageing is a product of a high metabolic rate".

3. **Become smarter.** The link between eating less and improved brain performance has been proven over and again. We are just wising up to this now but restricting diet to become more 'switched on' has been practised in many cultures for millennia. The great philosopher Pythagoras required his disciples to fast for 40 days. He claimed this would purify and clarify their minds sufficiently to grasp his profound teachings.

4. **Reduced insulin resistance.** Higher insulin resistance increases the risk of diabetes, obesity, and heart disease. Researchers in Japan have linked eating too quickly to insulin resistance.[102]

5. **Heartburn and gastroesophageal reflux.** Rapid eating can cause acid reflux.[103]

THE CLEANSE

Seriously, folks, this is a big one, and it's not at all hard to implement. The impact is also felt immediately. Here are the big-ticket items if you want to eat less, the ones that make a noticeable difference right away.

1. **Eat slower.** It takes the brain about fifteen to twenty minutes to tell you your stomach is full. If you are eating at a hundred miles an hour, a lot of food makes it to your belly before your brain can tell you to stop eating. If you eat slower, your brain will tell you that you are full by quelling your appetite before you have had a chance to eat too much.

2. **Chew more.** Chewing more can reduce your caloric intake by increasing the satisfaction you get from food. The more you chew the more you break food down, letting the gastric juices work more efficiently and allowing more nutrients and fluids to enter your gastrointestinal tract. You metabolise food more efficiently. The more you chew, the more saliva is produced. Saliva is the mouths natural defence against acid which causes tooth decay. Chewing also strengthens the jaw.

3. **Mindful eating.** This builds on the previous two items. Focus on the food you are eating, remove distractions, turn off the television, and leave your other electronic devices alone. We eat more when we are distracted. When you're eating slowly and chewing more, enjoy the taste, aroma, and texture of every bite. This will slow you down even more as the flavours linger in your mouth. Extended contact with your tastebuds will give you a better feeling of fullness. Buddha says to take it a step further and meditate on your food. Experience your food more intensively. Experience the pleasure of it.

4. **Fasting.** Clearly you eat less when you fast; you eat nothing. Cells in your body experience a stress reaction

with fasting as they do with exercise. This in turn extends your lifespan.[104] How? Your body burns fat instead of food-sourced glucose for fuel. Fat is a cleaner fuel than glucose, and burning it produces far fewer free radicals. Free radicals cause cell and DNA damage.

In addition, evidence suggests that when your body is provided with energy when it is not needed, such as before bed or when you are sleeping, cells leak electrons that react with oxygen and produce even more free radicals.[105] So by fasting you are promoting not only fat loss but also cell health. Poor cell health and cell dysfunction are linked with accelerated ageing and are behind many illnesses and diseases.

What, when, and how often you eat are key. Cell health is aided by eating real food, not eating several hours before sleeping to avoid excess glucose-based energy and fasting. Other benefits of fasting include a general reset and cleanse of the digestive system, greater mental clarity, cleansing of negative emotional patterns, and general feelings of lightness together with increased energy levels.

5. **Intermittent fasting.** Intermittent fasting is all about minimising free radical damage by teaching your body to burn fat for fuel by paying attention to the timing of your meals. During the first fourteen-to-sixteen hours of not eating, your body uses up all of its carbohydrate (glycogen) energy stores. After that it starts to use fat stores for energy.

The fast should last longer than this, but I don't like to fast longer than eighteen hours on a regular basis because I may start burning lean muscle mass for fuel by that time. So, with a sixteen-to-eighteen-hour fasting window, I have six to eight hours for eating my daily calories. I try to do this at least two days per week, although some would argue every day is better. This means I'll hold off on eating anything until around 10 a.m. and eat my last meal at 4 or 5 p.m. You can choose your own window of time. This reduces the body's habitual dependence on carbohydrates.

Another popular way to intermittently fast is, two days a week, only eat 25% of your usual calorie intake, but I find it too hard to work that out. All the benefits from producing fewer free radicals, lowered cancer risk, and greater fat loss have been demonstrated.[106] Scientists have also recently discovered that intermittent fasting can help regenerate stem cells, which are used by the body to renew itself.

Here are some simple tricks to help you eat less.

1. **Use smaller dishes**. This is nothing more than mental trickery. The same amount of food in a smaller plate just looks like more. Additionally, a full plate seems to look better to hungry eyes than a bigger plate that is half full.

2. **Serve 20% less**. This is the amount you can reduce your serving size without really noticing it. I've heard this referred to as the 'mindless margin'. If you plonk this reduced volume in a smaller dish, you'll notice it even less.

3. **Hide food.** The less you see, smell, and even hear food, the less you will be inclined to eat it. Do this by serving from the kitchen and leaving excess there, instead of on

the dining table. It also helps to keep food in cupboards, not out in the open.

4. **Avoid night-time snacks.** You'll never burn these calories, so if you must snack, eat healthy snacks or fruit or just drink water. Soda water does the trick for me.

5. **Drink water.** Before, during, and between helpings drink water to fill the gap instead of eating more food.

6. **Brush your teeth.** If your fangs are clean, you'll be less likely to want to affect that clean, minty feeling going on in your mouth.

––––––

We take eating for granted like we do breathing. But both these autonomous functions have moved centre stage for me since I started this cleanse. Be it breathing through meditation or eating through conscious eating, these are no longer just biological sideshows but two of the most important processes that go on in my day. In our fast food and fast eating world, we seem to have forgotten that food is not just a convenience but also one of the few things we actually need to survive. We seem to have forgotten where food comes from, how to grow it, how to respect it, and how to enjoy it. We even don't know what it is these days. I walk into a supermarket and am amazed at how much non-food is there. There's so much plastic and processed nonsense lining the shelves. I wonder how the hell we got to this point.

I am very picky about what I buy and what I prepare to eat. I cook only what I need, and I try to eat it as slowly and mindfully as possible. I eat with gratitude and thank the earth for sustaining me though each meal. I save food, money, and my health with this way of eating.

"Eat, drink, and be merry, for tomorrow we die." (Eccl 8:15 and Is 22:13)

———————

Section 3 – Conclusion

SUMMARY

Many of us humans consume too much. To a large degree we are products of our upbringing and our social and cultural environments. To consume too much is not only unnecessary but actually detrimental to our health. We consume goods as if on autopilot. The actual driver is an economic and marketing machine focused on infinite growth. Infinite growth is a dead-end street. This driver does not have human or planetary well-being in its instruction manual. We have evolved over the centuries and more so in recent decades to trust this driver. Folks, this driver is out of control. It is time to switch off the autopilot, take control of the wheel, and plot an evolutionary path that puts our well-being as the top priority.

Food is an obvious consumable to examine because it is one of the few things that we need to survive. Making informed, intelligent decisions about what we eat and disregarding the familiar status quo bends our otherwise dangerously off-course trajectory back to something that can be sustainable. This type of change must come from the bottom up, from the individual. It will not be delivered to your door by concerned governments or corporations because it goes against their most central tenet that we must consume more and grow infinitely.

RESULTS

Throughout the documentation of this process I realize that I have not avoided all personal, subjective ranting but this book does aim to be objective and factual. It had to be, given that it was spawned from my own desire to make effective, positive change. I've researched the major food and drinks that we consume according to what I've been told to eat and drink by history, custom, and marketing departments. It is from this research and my own personal experience that I have distilled the contents of this book. The experiment has come with a massive education. It has also been a lot of fun. I now know a great deal more about what I used to consume and what I now consume and why. Making the adjustments was not always easy. Real food is hard to find these days, especially in supermarkets. But the effort expended to source the food that is good for me has been paid back many times over.

Eating is now a central and conscious part of my life, and I can physically feel it when I veer off of the path. I falter from time to time, but in the main I know that going back to my old ways is not worth it. After completing the thirteen weeks of this cleanse I find myself weighing around fifteen kilograms less than before I started it. I feel distinctly healthier both physically and mentally, and my energy levels throughout the day are consistently higher. I also sleep at night now!

It's not just my health and my ecosystem that have reaped benefits from this cleanse. My wallet has as well. While it is true that for some categories of food and drink you might find that you need to spend more money, this is the exception rather than the rule. And besides, in these instances the foods themselves might cost a bit more, but if you consider the health costs (including your ecosystem's), they are probably cheaper in the long run. With more demand for real food, my hope is more supply will follow. With more supply we might expect downward pressures on prices.

Do It

My hope in documenting my findings and my experience is that it will inspire you to act and to do the Consumption Cleanse. You have nothing to lose and everything to gain including health, longevity, money, and time. This cleanse does require some effort, and while all of the changes in this cleanse may not stick forever, I can guarantee you that a lot of them will. And when they do, you will end up with a more evolved version of yourself.

And finally, as for what to do about the ducks, I'm afraid you are on you own.

About the Author

Michael Blue was born and educated (indoctrinated) in Brisbane, Australia. He is formally trained as an accountant and information technology specialist. Initially, his career was based in Australia, but from his mid-twenties, he spent as much time travelling and working abroad as he did in Australia. Throughout that time, he was self-educated as an escape artist.

He has been on the road living a simple, minimal life since June 2015 and until very recently called a big blue bus named Rosie his home. That bus, which provided transport, a place to sleep, cook, contemplate, and write, would most commonly be found adrift somewhere in Sumatra, Indonesia. There is no plan and no map, but a driving desire to live outside of the consumption society and live in a way that prioritises physical and mental well-being, integration with the natural world, and human community and creativity.

You can connect with Michael at:

Website: https://thelifeadrift.com/

Email: thelifeadrift@gmail.com

Facebook: https://www.facebook.com/thelifeadrift/

Instagram: https://www.instagram.com/blueyadrift/

Twitter: https://twitter.com/MikeBlue111

Other Titles

Have you ever asked yourself if our ideas about success are all they're made out to be? Do you ever wonder if work and pursuit of money and material possessions are ALL THERE IS to life? *The Anatomy of Escape*.

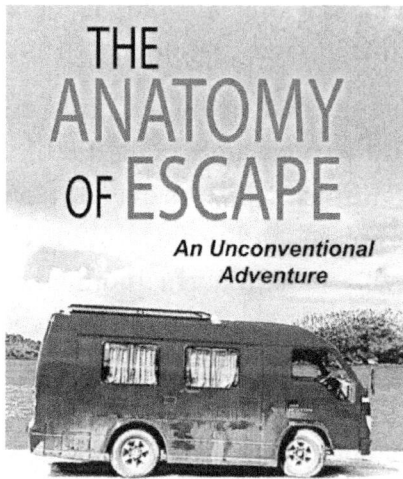

THE
ANATOMY
OF ESCAPE

An Unconventional Adventure

Michael Blue

For twenty years, the author, an accountant trapped on the corporate treadmill, contemplated these questions. Now he lives in a bus in the dense jungles of Northern Sumatra. This is his idea of freedom. He is a fugitive of an unusual kind, an escapee from the work-consume-die hamster wheel. He has a simple existence without much use for work or money. *The Anatomy of Escape* is the story of how he got there.

Get it on Amazon now: http://a.co/9uVCksa

Reviews are Gold to Authors

If you enjoyed this book and would like to help, then you could think about leaving a review on Amazon, Goodreads, or anywhere else that readers visit. The most important part of how well a book sells is how many positive reviews it has, so if you leave me one then you are directly helping me to continue on this journey as a writer. It will only take a few minutes of your time. Thanks in advance to anyone who does. It means a lot.

End Notes

[1] William Rees. University of British Columbia. Retrieved from http://www.globalissues.org/article/238/effects-of-consumerism.

[2] European Association for the Study of Obesity. "Obesity Facts and Figures." Retrieved from http://easo.org/education-portal/obesity-facts-figures; World Health Organization. "Global Health Authority (GHO) Data." Retrieved from http://www.who.int/gho/ncd/mortality_morbidity/cvd/en; World Health Organization. "The Top 10 Causes of Death." Retrieved from http://www.who.int/mediacentre/factsheets/fs310/en.

[3] Damon Gameau. *That Sugar Film.* Retrieved from http://www.thatsugarfilm.com/film.

[4] Kris Gunnars. "Top 10 Reasons to Avoid Sugar as If Your Life Depended on It." Retrieved from http://authoritynutrition.com/9-reasons-to-avoid-sugar.

[5] Monell Chemical Senses Center, University of Pennsylvania. "Dietary Fructose Reduces Circulating Insulin and Leptin, Attenuates Postprandial Suppression of Ghrelin, and Increases Triglycerides in Women. Retrieved from http://www.ncbi.nlm.nih.gov/pubmed/15181085; Yale University School of Medicine. "Effects of Fructose vs. Glucose on Regional Cerebral Blood Flow in Brain Regions Involved with Appetite and Reward Pathways." Retrieved from http://www.ncbi.nlm.nih.gov/pubmed/23280226.

[6] A. Breeze Harper. *Sistah Vegan.* New York, NY: Lantern Books, 2010, p. 24.

[7] Brown, K. et al. "Diet-Induced Dysbiosis of the Intestinal Microbiota and the Effects on Immunity and Disease." Nutrients. 4(8).

[8] Wikipedia. "List of Countries by Beer Consumption per Capita." Retrieved from https://en.wikipedia.org/wiki/List_of_countries_by_beer_consumpti

on_per_capita.

[9] N. Shay, M. Okla, I. Kang, D. M. Kim, V. Gourineni, and S. Chung. "Ellagic Acid Modulates Lipid Accumulation in Primary Human Adipocytes and Human Hepatoma Huh7 Cells via Discrete Mechanisms." *The Journal of Nutritional Biochemistry*, 2015 Jan; 26(1):82-90.

[10] Thinkinghumanity.com. "A Glass of Red Wine Can Replace an Hour of Exercising According to New Study." Retrieved from http://www.thinkinghumanity.com/2015/12/a-glass-of-red-wine-can-replace-an-hour-of-exercising-according-to-new-study.html.

[11] Michael Moss. *Salt, Sugar, Fat: How the Food Giants Hooked Us.* New York, NY: Random House, 2013.

[12] Eleni Roumeliotou. "Addiction to Junk Food: More Than Meets the Eye." Retrieved from http://www.wakingtimes.com/2013/04/08/addiction-to-junk-food-more-than-meets-the-eye.

[13] UNICEF. "Breastfeeding and complimentary feeding." Retrieved from http://www.unicef.org/nutrition/index_breastfeeding.html.

[14] GMOInside.org. "Abbot, Mead Johnson, and Nestlé: Our Babies Deserve Better than GMOs!" Retrieved from http://action.greenamerica.org/p/dia/action/public/?action_KEY=1 0597.

[15] Jordan Light. "Melamine Traces Found in Samples of US Infant Formula." Retrieved from http://blogs.scientificamerican.com/news-blog/melamine-traces-found-in-samples-of-2008-11-26.

[16] Daniella Silva. "Lawsuit Claims Purina's Beneful Is Poisoning, Killing Dogs." Retrieved from http://www.nbcnews.com/news/us-news/lawsuit-claims-purinas-beneful-poisoning-killing-dogs-n312176.

[17] Charley Cameron. "How Nestle Is Pillaging California's Water in the 4th Year of the State's Worst Drought." Retrieved from http://inhabitat.com/how-nestle-is-pillaging-californias-water-in-

the-4th-year-of-the-states-worst-drought.

[18] Ian James. "Little Oversight as Nestle Taps Morongo Reservation Water." Retrieved from http://www.desertsun.com/story/news/environment/2014/07/12/nestle-arrowhead-tapping-water/12589267.

[19] Worldcrunch. "Poisoning the Well? Nestle Accused of Exploiting Water Supplies for Bottled Brands." Retrieved from http://www.worldcrunch.com/poisoning-well-nestl-accused-exploiting-water-supplies-bottled-brands/business-finance/poisoning-the-well-nestl-accused-of-exploiting-water-supplies-for-bottled-brands/c2s4503/#.UXEDk7VTCtY.

[20] Miki Mistrati and U. Roberto Romano. "The Dark Side of Chocolate." Retrieved from https://www.youtube.com/watch?v=7Vfbv6hNeng.

[21] Matthew Boesler. "Bottled Water Costs 2000 Times as Much as Tap Water." Retrieved from http://www.businessinsider.com/bottled-water-costs-2000x-more-than-tap-2013-7?IR=T&r=US&IR=T.

[22] Waking Times. "High Fructose Corn Syrup Now Hidden Under a New Name." Retrieved from http://www.wakingtimes.com/2015/12/09/high-fructose-corn-syrup-now-hidden-under-a-new-name.

23 Hector D, Rangan A, Louie J, Flood V, Gill T. "Soft drinks, weight status and health: a review." Retrieved from http://ro.uow.edu.au/cgi/viewcontent.cgi?article=1317&context=hbspapers

[24] Chistina Sarich. "6 FDA Approved Foods That Are Banned in Other Counties." Retrieved from http://consciouslifenews.com/6-fda-approved-foods-banned-other-countries/1185122.

[25] Plosone.org."Identification of Putative Steroid Receptor Antagonists in Bottled Water: Combining Bioassays and High-Resolution Mass Spectrometry." Retrieved from

http://journals.plos.org/plosone/article?id=10.1371/journal.pone.0 072472.

26 Pacific Institute. "Integrity of Science: Bottled Water and Energy Factsheet: Getting to 17 Million Barrels." Retrieved from http://pacinst.org/publication/bottled-water-fact-sheet/.

27 The Story of Stuff Project. "The Story of Bottled Water". Retrieved from http://storyofstuff.org/movies/story-of-bottled-water/

28 E.g. Business Insider. "11 Incredible Facts About The Global Coffee Industry." Retrieved from http://www.businessinsider.com/facts-about-the-coffee-industry-2011-11?IR=T&r=US&IR=T#after-crude-oil-coffee-is-the-most-sought-commodity-in-the-world-1 and Mark Pendergrast. "Uncommon Grounds: The History of Coffee and How It Transformed Our World". (Basic Books, 1999)

29 CaffeineInformer.com. "Caffeine Absorption." Retrieved from http://www.caffeineinformer.com/caffeine-absorption.

30 Miguel A. Hernán, et al. "A Meta-Analysis of Coffee Drinking, Cigarette Smoking, and the Risk of Parkinson's Disease." *Annals of Neurology,* 52(3), 276–284.

31 Miguel A. Hernán, et al. "A Meta-Analysis of Coffee Drinking, Cigarette Smoking, and the Risk of Parkinson's Disease." *Annals of Neurology,* 52(3), 276–284.

32 Anthony P. Winston, Elizabeth Hardwick, and Neema Jaberi. "Neuropsychiatric Effects of Caffeine." *Advances in Psychiatric Treatment* 11(6), 432–439.

33 J. Snel. "Effects of Caffeine on Sleep and Cognition." Retrieved from http://www.ncbi.nlm.nih.gov/pubmed/21531247.

34 M. S. Butt and M. T. Sultan. "Coffee and Its Consumption: Benefits and Risks." *Critical Reviews in Food Science and Nutrition* 51(4): 363–373.

35 Wikipedia. "Economics of Coffee." Retrieved from

https://en.wikipedia.org/wiki/Economics_of_coffee

[36] Teeccino Product Website. "Non-Acidic." Retrieved from http://teeccino.com/about/39/Non-Acidic.html

[37] Salim M. Ali. "Meat: The Opium of the 21st Century." Norderstedt Books on Demand, 2015.

[38] Slowfood.com. "How Much Meat Do We Eat?." Retrieved from http://www.slowfood.com/slowmeat/en/the-meat-we-eat/how-much-meat-do-we-eat.

[39] David Goldstein. "Up Close: A Beef with Dairy." KCAL, 30 May 2002.

[40] Mercy for Animals. "From Farm to Fridge—The Truth about Meat Production." Retrieved from https://www.youtube.com/watch?v=THIODWTqx5E.

[41] Michael Gregor. "Do Vegetarians Get Enough Protein?" Retrieved from http://nutritionfacts.org/video/do-vegetarians-get-enough-protein.

[42] Harper, p. 24.

[43] Kip Andersen and Keegan Kuhn, *Cowspiracy: The Sustainability Secret*. Retrieved from http://www.cowspiracy.com.

[44] AllCreatures.org. "15 Reasons to Stop Eating Meat." Retrieved from http://www.all-creatures.org/articles/env-15.html

[45] Kai Olsen-Sawyer. "Meat's Large Water Footprint: Why Raising Livestock and Poultry for Meat Is So Resource-Intensive." Retrieved from http://foodtank.com/news/2013/12/why-meat-eats-resources.

[46] Deborah Wilson. "Eating Meat Is Linked to Obesity." Retrieved from http://www.peta.org/issues/animals-used-for-food/obesity.

[47] Sarah Glynn. "Vegetarians Live Longer than Meat-Eaters." Retrieved from http://www.medicalnewstoday.com/articles/261382.php.

[48] Mark Devries. *Speciesism: The Movie*. Retrieved from http://speciesismthemovie.com.

[49] Harvard Health Publications. "Glycemic Index and Glycemic Load for 100+ Foods." Retrieved from http://www.health.harvard.edu/diseases-and-conditions/glycemic_index_and_glycemic_load_for_100_foods.

[50] ARJUN WALIA. "LOBBYIST SAYS MONSANTO'S ROUNDUP IS SAFE TO DRINK – WHEN OFFERED A GLASS HE FREAKS OUT." Retrieved from http://www.collective-evolution.com/2016/01/22/lobbyist-says-monsantos-roundup-is-safe-to-drink-when-offered-a-glass-he-freaks-out/

[51] Sarah Pope. "Monsanto's Roundup Responsible for Skyrocketing Rates of Celiac Disease, Gluten Intolerance and Other Wheat-Related Illnesses." Retrieved from http://www.globalresearch.ca/monsantos-roundup-responsible-for-skyrocketing-rates-of-celiac-disease-gluten-intolerance-and-other-wheat-related-illnesses/5419461.

[52] Nga M. Lau, et al. "Markers of Celiac Disease and Gluten Sensitivity in Children with Autism." Retrieved from http://journals.plos.org/plosone/article?id=10.1371/journal.pone.0066155.

[53] The Fifth Estate. "The War on Wheat". Retrieved from https://www.youtube.com/watch?v=eO3cIrNEuIc

54 Michael Greger. "Cancer Risk from French Fries". Retrieved from

http://nutritionfacts.org/video/cancer-risk-from-french-fries/

[55] Y. Srivastava and A. D. Semwal. "A Study on Monitoring of Frying Performance and Oxidative Stability of Virgin Coconut Oil (VCO) During Continuous/Prolonged Deep Fat Frying Process Using Chemical and FTIR Spectroscopy". Retrieved from http://www.ncbi.nlm.nih.gov/pubmed/25694709.

[56] ISAAA. "Beyond Promises: Top 10 Facts about Biotech/GM Crops

in 2014." Retrieved from
http://www.isaaa.org/resources/publications/biotech_booklets/top
_10_facts/download/Top%2010%20Facts%20Booklet.pdf.

[57] Dr Mae-Wan Ho. "Bangladesh: Farmers say No to Genetically Modified Vegetables." The Ecologist, 2014

[58] *Natural News.* "Genetically modified eggplant a massive failure in Bangladesh as crops fail for second year in a row." Retrieved from http://www.naturalnews.com/052079_GM_eggplant_Bt_brinjal_crop _failures.html.

[59] Micha Peled. "Bitter Seeds." Retrieved from https://www.youtube.com/watch?v=QZtKB_KuASc.

[60] Union of Concerned Scientists. "Failure to Yield—Evaluating the Performance of Genetically Engineered Crops." Retrieved from http://www.ucsusa.org/sites/default/files/legacy/assets/document s/food_and_agriculture/failure-to-yield.pdf.

[61] Pushpa M. Bhargava. "US Is Trying to Control Our Food Production." *Hindustan Times.* August 7, 2014 Retrieved from http://www.hindustantimes.com/comment/analysis/us-is-trying-to-control-our-food-production/article1-1249456.aspx.

[62] Steven M. Druker. *Altered Genes, Twisted Truth.* Fairfield, IA: Clear River Press, 2015.

[63] Sa´ndorSpisa´k, et al. "Complete Genes May Pass from Food to Human Blood." Retrieved from http://www.gmoevidence.com/wp-content/uploads/2013/08/journal.pone_.0069805.pdf.

[64] Channa Jayasumana, et al. "Glyphosate, Hard Water and Nephrotoxic Metals: Are They the Culprits Behind the Epidemic of Chronic Kidney Disease of Unknown Etiology in Sri Lanka?" *International Journal of Environ. Research and Public Health.* 11(2), 2125–2147.

[65] Judy Camen. "Evidence of GMO Harm in Pig Study." Retrieved from http://gmojudycarman.org/new-study-shows-that-animals-are-seriously-harmed-by-gm-feed.

[66] Jeffrey Dach. "GMO Food Scandal." Retrieved from http://www.drdach.com/Dr_Dach_on_GMO_Food_Scandal.html.

[67] GreenMedInfo. "44 Reasons to Ban or Label GMOs." Retrieved from http://www.greenmedinfo.com/blog/44-reasons-ban-or-label-gmos.

[68] Gilles-Eric Seralini. "Long-Term Toxicity of a Roundup Herbicide and a Roundup-Tolerant Genetically Modified Maize." *Food and Chemical Toxicology*, Volume 69, July 2014, Pages 357-359.

[69] Steve Volk. "Suspended USDA Researcher Alleges Agency Tried to Block His Research into Harmful Effects of Pesticides on Bees, Butterflies." *Washington Post*. October 28, 2015.

[70] Kim Jeong-su. "More Genetically Modified Crops Found Growing in South Korea." Retrieved from http://www.hani.co.kr/arti/english_edition/e_business/590585.htm l.

[71] UN FAO. "Global Dairy Sector: Status and Trends." Retrieved from http://www.fao.org/docrep/012/i1522e/i1522e02.pdf.

[72] T. Colin Campbell and Thomas M. Campbell. The China Study: The Most Comprehensive Study of Nutrition Ever Conducted and the Startling Implications for Diet, Weight Loss and Long-term Health. Dallas, TX: BenBella Books, 2004.

[73] Harvard T. H. Chan School of Public Health. "Calcium and Milk: What's Best for Your Bones and Health?" Retrieved from http://www.hsph.harvard.edu/nutritionsource/calcium-full-story.

[74] R. G. Cumming and R. J. Klineberg. "Case-Control Study of Risk Factors for Hip Fractures in the Elderly." *American Journal of Epidemiology*, 139(5), 493–503.

[75] D. M. Swallow. "Genetics of Lactase Persistence and Lactose Intolerance." *National Center for Biotechnology Information*, 37, 197–219.

[76] Bethany A. Pribila, et. al. "Improved Lactose Digestion and

Intolerance Among African-American Adolescent Girls Fed a Dairy Rich-Diet." Journal of the Academy of Nutrition and Dietetics, 100, 524-528. Retrieved from http://www.andjrnl.org/article/S0002-8223(00)00162-0/abstract

[77] H. Elsa, et al. "Diet and Acne: A Review of the Evidence." Retrieved from http://onlinelibrary.wiley.com/doi/10.1111/j.1365-4632.2009.04002.x/full

[78] R. Kaaks. "Nutrition, Insulin, IGF-1 Metabolism and Cancer Risk: A Summary of Epidemiological Evidence." Retrieved from shttp://www.ncbi.nlm.nih.gov/pubmed/15562834.

[79] Susanna C Larsson, et al. "Milk and Lactose Intakes and Ovarian Cancer Risk in the Swedish Mammography Cohort1, 2, 3." Retrieved from http://ajcn.nutrition.org/content/80/5/1353.abstract.

[80] Erin Janus. "DAIRY IS F**KING SCARY! The industry explained in 5 minutes." Retrieved from https://www.youtube.com/watch?v=UcN7SGGoCNI

[81] Kristin Canty. *Farmageddon*. 2011. Retrieved from https://www.youtube.com/watch?v=2rLe0zMRLOs.

[82] Academy of Culinary Nutrition. "20 Best Dairy-Free Ice Cream Recipes." Retrieve from http://www.culinarynutrition.com/20-best-dairy-free-ice-cream-recipes/

[83] The Safina Center. "Seafoods". Retrieved from http://safinacenter.org/files/Seafood_Guide.pdf

[84] Michael D'Orso and Ted Danson. *Oceana: Our Endangered Oceans and What We Can Do to Save Them*. New York, NY: Rodale Books, 2011.

[85] National Geographic Society. *Pristine Seas—Overfishing*. Retrieved from http://ocean.nationalgeographic.com/ocean/explore/pristine-seas/critical-issues-overfishing.

[86] Oceana. "Responsible Fishing Stopping Overfishing." Retrieved

from http://oceana.org/our-campaigns/promote_responsible_fishing/campaign.

[87] UN FAO. "The State of World Fisheries and Aquaculture." Retrieved from http://www.fao.org/docrep/013/i1820e/i1820e00.htm.

[88] Kistine Lofgren. "35 Facts That Will Make You Never Want to Eat Fish Again." Retrieved from http://inhabitat.com/35-facts-that-will-make-you-never-want-to-eat-fish-again.

[89] Nicole Greenfield. *The Smart Seafood Buying Guide.* Retrieved from https://www.nrdc.org/stories/smart-seafood-buying-guide.

[90] Alex Roslin. "Canada: Fish Eaters Threatened by Fukushima Radiation." *The Vancouver Sun*, 16 Jan 2012.

[91] Washingtons Blog. "Absolutely Every One—15 Out of 15—Bluefin Tuna Tested in California Waters Contaminated with Fukushima Radiation." Retrieved from http://www.washingtonsblog.com/2012/05/absolutely-every-one-of-the-15-bluefin-tuna-tested-in-california-waters-contaminated-with-fukushima-radiation.html.

[92] Nicolas Daniel. *Fillet Oh Fish.* Retrieved from https://www.youtube.com/watch?v=MgrFXN4d1Jc.

[93] U.S. Food & Drug Administration. "Overview of Food Ingredients, Additives & Colors." Retrieved from http://www.fda.gov/Food/IngredientsPackagingLabeling/FoodAdditivesIngredients/ucm094211.htm

[94] Kenneth Bock and Cameron Stauth. "Healing the New Childhood Epidemics: Autism, ADHD, Asthma, and Allergies: The Groundbreaking Program for the 4-A Disorders." New York, NY: Ballantine Books, 2008.

[95] Center for Science in the Public Interest. "Summary of Studies on Food Dyes." Retrieved from http://cspinet.org/new/pdf/dyes-problem-table.pdf.

[96] Northern Allergy Center. "Hyperactive Children's Support Group's Guide to Food Additives." Retrieved from http://nac.allergyforum.com/additives/colors100-181.htm.

[97] Akiko Shimada, et. al. "Headache and Mechanical Sensitization of Human Pericranial Muscles after Repeated Intake of Monosodium Glutamate (MSG)." Retrieved from http://www.ncbi.nlm.nih.gov/pmc/articles/PMC3606962/#!po=42.5000.

[98] Wikipedia. "Sodium Nitrite." Retrieved from https://en.wikipedia.org/wiki/Sodium_nitrite

[99] The UK Food Guide. "Sulphur Dioxide." Retrieved from http://www.ukfoodguide.net/e220.htm

[100] Shawn Radcliffe. "KEEP YOUR HEART YOUNG BY EATING LESS". Retrieved from http://www.mensfitness.com/nutrition/what-to-eat/keep-your-heart-young-by-eating-less

[101] David Tenenbaum. "Monkey caloric restriction study shows big benefit; contradicts earlier study." Retrieved from http://news.wisc.edu/monkey-caloric-restriction-study-shows-big-benefit-contradicts-earlier-study/

[102] R. Otsuka, et al. "Eating Fast Leads to Insulin Resistance: Findings in Middle-Aged Japanese Men and Women. *Preventative Medicine*, 2008 Feb;46(2):154-9.

[103] S. M. Wildi, and Tutuian R. Castell. "The Influence of Rapid Food Intake on Postprandial Reflux: Studies in Healthy Volunteers. *American Journal of Gastroenterology*, 99(9), 1645–51.

[104] Mercola. "Studies Show Eating More Slowly Benefits Your Health and Waistline." Retrieved from http://fitness.mercola.com/sites/fitness/archive/2016/03/25/health-benefits-fasting.aspx#_edn1

[105] Ibid.

[106] Ibid.

Printed in Great Britain
by Amazon

34859366R00121